Working with Ethnic Minorities and Across Cultures in Western Child Protection Systems

T0186330

Multiculturalism in Western countries continues to grow, but responsiveness to it with culturally sensitive research, policy and practice has been slower to develop. This lag could be accused of enabling institutional racism – that is, culturally insensitive practices and policies can cause or perpetuate harm to non-mainstream children and families, the very thing that child protection systems are set up to address. Thus, it is critical that the field has a resource that clearly and comprehensively outlines the characteristics of cultural competency in the child protection system when working with ethnic minorities and across both mainstream and non-mainstream cultures, so as to equally protect the safety of all children.

Unlike previous research, this book addresses discrete and relevant practice issues – how to work effectively with interpreters, whether or not to match caseworkers and clients based on ethnic background and what to consider when making plans for children in the out-of-home care (OOHC) system – with best practice guidelines. This book will be required reading for all social work students, academics and practitioners whose work engages with issues of cultural competency.

Pooja Sawrikar is Postdoctoral Fellow in Social Policy at Griffith University, Australia.

Contemporary Social Work Studies

Series Editors:
Lucy Jordan, The University of Hong Kong, China
Patrick O'Leary, Griffith University, Australia

Contemporary Social Work Studies is a series disseminating high quality new research and scholarship in the discipline and profession of social work. The series promotes critical engagement with contemporary issues relevant across the social work community and captures the diversity of interests currently evident at national, international and local levels.

Other titles in the series include:

Revitalising Communities in a Globalising World
Practices of Power and Resistance
Edited by Lena Dominelli

Social Work in a Corporate Era
Practices of Power and Resistance
Edited by Linda Davies and Peter Leonard

Reflecting on Social Work - Discipline and Profession
Edited by Robin Lovelock, Karen Lyons and Jackie Powell

Broadening Horizons
International Exchanges in Social Work
Edited by Lena Dominelli and Wanda Thomas Bernard

Beyond Racial Divides
Ethnicities in Social Work Practice
Edited by Lena Dominelli, Walter Lorenz and Haluk Soydan

Working with Ethnic Minorities and Across Cultures in Western Child Protection Systems
Pooja Sawrikar

Working with Ethnic Minorities and Across Cultures in Western Child Protection Systems

Pooja Sawrikar

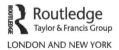
Routledge
Taylor & Francis Group

LONDON AND NEW YORK

First published 2017
by Routledge
2 Park Square, Milton Park, Abingdon, Oxon OX14 4RN

and by Routledge
711 Third Avenue, New York, NY 10017

Routledge is an imprint of the Taylor & Francis Group, an informa business

British Library Cataloguing in Publication Data
A catalogue record for this book is available from the British Library

Library of Congress Cataloging in Publication Data
A catalog record for this book has been requested

ISBN: 978-1-138-22583-1 (hbk)
ISBN: 978-1-138-22584-8 (pbk)
ISBN: 978-1-315-39314-8 (ebk)

Typeset in Times New Roman
by Saxon Graphics Ltd, Derby

Printed and bound in Great Britain by Ashford Colour Press Ltd.

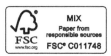

To my parents for investing in my foundations, and to my husband for investing in our son while I wrote this book.

Contents

Illustrations

Tables

Figures

Acknowledgements

This book is based on a Postdoctoral Fellowship that was jointly funded by the New South Wales (NSW) Department of Family and Community Services (FaCS) in Australia and the Social Policy Research Centre (SPRC) at the University of New South Wales (UNSW) also in Australia. I would like to sincerely thank them both for providing the opportunity to conduct this study. In addition, I wish to acknowledge contributions from the FaCS Steering Committee for their ongoing input and advice on the project design and its progress, including members of FaCS' Multicultural Services Unit (MSU), Parenting Research Centre (PRC), Information Management Branch (IMB) and local Community Service Centres (CSCs) – Gloria Bromley, (the late) Mary Dimech, Fay Kitto, Mary Labbad, Paul Mortimer, Eileen Ross, Julie Young, Peter Walsh, Johanna Watson and Angela White. I would also like to thank Professor Ilan Katz and Ryan Gleeson from SPRC for providing mentoring and research assistance, respectively. I want to also thank all the people I worked with at Ashgate Publishing Ltd – Claire Jarvis, Lianne Sherlock, Amanda Buxton, Patrick O'Leary, Emma Chappell, Anna Dolan, Sarah Cheeseman, Rosie McDonald and Shannon Kneis – for their kind support and constructive feedback throughout the entire publishing process. Perhaps most importantly, however, I would like to thank the caseworkers and case managers in the ten CSCs that took part in this study (whom I have not named here, partly because there are so many, but mostly to protect their anonymity). They assisted in various aspects of the project (most especially the recruitment of family interviewees), but they also took the time to share their passion, knowledge and humour in 'corridor conversations' that helped add depth and texture to the formal part of the study. In short, many people have inspired and assisted in the production of the contents of this book – to them, thank you.

This research has been undertaken with assistance from the NSW Department of Community Services. However, the information and views contained in this study do not necessarily, or at all, reflect the views or information held by the NSW Government, the Minister for Community Services or the Department.

Common abbreviations

AOD   Alcohol or Other Drug Issue
AVO   Apprehended Violence Order
CALD   Culturally and Linguistically Diverse
CP   Child Protection
CSC   (FaCS') Community Service Centre
CW   Caseworker
DoCS[1] Department of Community Services
DV   Domestic Violence
FaCS   Department of Family and Community Services
MH   Mental Health
NESB   Non-English Speaking Background
NF   Natural Father
NM   Natural Mother
OOHC   Out-of-Home Care
PR   Parental Responsibility
ROH[2] Risk of Harm
SC   Subject Child

Notes

1 At the time the study was conducted, the New South Wales (NSW) Department of Family and Community Services (FaCS) was known as the NSW Department of Community Services (DoCS). The name change occurred in 2010.
2 At the time the study was conducted, risk of harm (ROH) rather than risk of *significant* harm (ROSH) was used in assessments and substantiations of maltreatment. In 2014 FaCS changed its policy to investigate only children that met ROSH, leaving (non-statutory) non-government organisations (NGOs) to investigate and support families that fell under this threshold.

Introduction
What is in this book and who should use it

Statutory and non-statutory child protection workers, providers of services related to child and family welfare, policy makers responsible for child safety, social work students and academic researchers that are empathic to the importance of culture come from all walks of life; they do not just emerge from those who are of ethnic minority backgrounds themselves. Several white, English speaking practitioners and policy makers understand just how crucial it is to give the right amount and right kind of space to this topic, and actively advocate for it, to ensure that all children are safe and equally safe. While this book has the aforementioned groups as its key target audiences, there is a common risk with any such book that is specific in focus and cause – it ends up 'preaching to the converted' (though it is not assumed that everyone will agree with all aspects of the book). It is for this reason that the target groups for this book are in fact *all* child protection workers, service providers in child and family welfare, policy makers responsible for child safety and academics in the field. It is also intended that this book be used by ethnic minority children and families themselves as a reference for the representation of their voices, experiences and needs. The importance of culture in the protection of children is so fundamental that knowledge should be in the hands of all key stakeholders and peak bodies, not just in the few who care.

Indeed, multiculturalism in Western countries is a fact (whether some like it or not), and it is certainly not on the demise. The lag in responsiveness to changing population demographics with culturally sensitive research, policy and practice could be benignly attributed to small sample sizes in the past or it could be attributed to a more aggressive accusation of enabling institutional racism. Even if the reason lies somewhere in the middle, action and voices are needed. It cannot be assumed that just because migrants of non-English speaking background (NESB) collectively comprise the minority of a Western nation's population, their cultures then are minor in value and importance. Protecting the right of all groups to preserve and celebrate their culture and cultural differences is in fact the only way a child can be truly safe from harm and all children can be truly safe from harm equally – this includes harm from family perpetrators as well as harm from child protection systems, which can be perpetrators of child abuse and neglect themselves if they fail to protect children. Thus, culture is an issue for every child in every multicultural society, and anyone who is involved in child safety in a

Western country, in which social power is unequally distributed and ethnic minorities have significantly less of it than their mainstream counterparts, should be familiar with and mindful of the concepts and issues raised in this book.

This book does not claim to be exhaustive because it is difficult to offer such a thing on such a vast and complex topic, but great effort has been made to at least try. This book is based on a large-scale, three-year study that was conducted to explore culturally appropriate child protection service delivery with culturally and linguistically diverse (CALD) children and families, funded under a competitively awarded Postdoctoral Fellowship by the New South Wales (NSW) Department of Family and Community Services (FaCS, then known as the NSW Department of Community Services or DoCS – the state's statutory child protection authority) and the Social Policy Research Centre (SPRC) at the University of New South Wales (UNSW) in Australia. The study was comprised of three detailed and thorough stages: (1) a literature review, (2) 120 case file reviews and (3) 46 interviews. Thus, it was able to triangulate both quantitative and qualitative methodologies, and mixed methods approaches to theory, data collection and data analysis all help improve the representativeness of a study's findings.

Detailed information on the three stages can be found in the chapter on the study's methodology (e.g. breakdown of case files by age, sex and cultural background, details of interviewees, etc.). This will allow a reader to understand the scope of the book's material, but also refer to any section of it for more precise information on the way the study was conducted and sample demographics. These details are important for contextualising the study's results but ultimately, it is the themes that the results point to that form the bulk of this book. These themes are fleshed out in Parts I, II and III where there is greater focus on theoretical issues, practice issues and models for good practice.

The literature review and qualitative interviews primarily form the basis of Part I of this book, which aims to do two things. First, it aims to describe the client group of interest and second, it sets the theoretical backdrop as to why culture is an important variable to consider in child protection work in Western countries.

Chapter 1 begins with an assumption that the reader does not have basic information or knowledge about ethnic minorities in Western countries. This does not reflect a belief that Western academics, service providers, social work students and policy makers are not 'in the know' of such matters. It is simply an assurance that all readers – no matter where they may be on their journey of letting the importance of culture into their work practice – get all the relevant information they may need. In short, this chapter outlines how ethnic minorities – also referred to in the literature as those of NESB and the CALD – have some things in common with each other: typically, English is not the main language, collectivist values that protect the family name and privacy are common and a host of experiences emerge as a result of being a migrant – displaced sense of identity, racism and discrimination, intergenerational conflict, lack of awareness of child protection systems, social isolation, socio-economic disadvantage, etc. This information helps frame the client group – who they are and what they typically experience as an ethnic minority in a Western country – even before they enter the child protection system, but also while in it.

Chapter 2 is particularly dense. It outlines why culture is critical in child protection matters and their relationship is complex. In brief, here, it has to do with two things – accuracy in assessments and parity in assessments – but this chapter additionally argues that the only way all children from different cultural backgrounds can be protected equally is through accurate risk of harm assessments. Thus, parity in the protection of children across cultures is not in having one ethnocentric child protection law disguised as an absolute standard – such a colour-blind approach leaves children from some groups vulnerable either to abuse and neglect from family perpetrators or to abuse and neglect from child protection systems. Instead, it is in the full and serious consideration of culture for all children because culture frames our understanding and definitions of abuse and neglect, and so accurate assessments of abuse and neglect require consideration of culture. Taking culture into account in the right way and to the right extent: (i) prevents institutional racism – where ethnocentric tools of assessment are used to judge the safety of ethnic minority children and possibly lead to inaccurate allegations of maltreatment (false positives), and (ii) avoids mistaking maltreatment as culturally acceptable (false negatives), exacerbated by defensiveness in families struggling to protect the safety of their culture, and fear of being labelled racist in white caseworkers.

In other words, some sort of balance is required between 'cultural absolutism' – the position that culture does not need to be considered in child protection matters – and 'cultural relativism' – the position that culture is so important it could trump child safety. In practical terms, this means having one child protection law driven above all else by a child-centred philosophy, a need for accuracy, an holistic approach (including the need for a child's right to be cared for by their family) and a focus more on outcomes for children than the intent of the caregiver. It also requires child protection caseworkers and systems being fully educated on and aware of the pitfalls of cultural absolutism and relativism and accepting the subjectivity that comes with applying that knowledge on a case-by-case basis. These all help ensure that individualistic and collectivist conceptualisations of family and its role in child-rearing are equally valued, and that the minority status of non-mainstream groups is acknowledged in the diagnosis of maltreatment and the tailored delivery of intervention; all children can be said to be equally protected from harm regardless of their cultural background when a child's cultural needs are neither over-stated nor overlooked.

In Part II, the reader will find a number of chapters that address specific issues that are likely to arise in practice. In Chapter 3, it is now assumed that a child has entered the child protection system, (and the chapters from here on then relate to various aspects of this). It uses data from the case file reviews to report on the frequency of reports for physical abuse, sexual abuse, emotional abuse, inadequate supervision, neglect of basic needs and educational neglect for six cultural groups in the state of NSW in Australia. These six groups are Chinese, Vietnamese, Pacific Islander (Samoan and Tongan), Lebanese, Aboriginal and Anglo Saxon/Celtic (henceforth Anglo). The first four of these groups are considered to be 'ethnic minorities', Aboriginals are considered First Nation people and Anglos are considered to be the mainstream. While other Western countries like the United States of America (USA), the United Kingdom (UK), Canada and New Zealand (NZ) have different demographic profiles to Australia, it can be argued that the experiences and processes that occur for ethnic minorities (and First Nation and mainstream people) are similar enough to yield this Australian data transferable to, or representative of, other comparable Western countries. The main finding was that reports of physical abuse are higher in ethnic minorities, and reports of sexual abuse are higher in First Nation and mainstream groups. This chapter also uses case file data to make the point that maltreated children, regardless of their cultural background, are at risk of similar outcomes; the two most common being behavioural issues and mental health issues.

Chapter 4 addresses, perhaps, one of the most important issues in this field of practice and which emerged from the case file data in Chapter 3 by triangulating it with the literature review and data from the qualitative interviews: why are reports of physical abuse higher in ethnic minorities and reports of sexual abuse higher in Aboriginal and Anglo groups, and does culture have something to do with these cross-cultural differences? In brief, physical discipline is generally an acceptable form of parenting in collective cultures (which ethnic minorities tend to be), and physical discipline may be deemed abusive by child protection workers in Western countries, in which case there are higher reports of physical abuse for these groups. However, because culture is entwined with parenting and discipline – being normative, acceptable and of value – this area of engagement with ethnic minority families particularly requires cultural awareness, sensitivity and competency so that ethnic minorities do not feel that their culture is being disrespected; that is, education to increase insight on the harmful effects of physical discipline is seen as a culturally appropriate 'first step' of engagement. In comparison to physical abuse, culture is not entwined with a diagnosis of sexual abuse – since no culture condones it – but it may still be tied in with culture in the way that it is addressed with families by caseworkers, with family name and privacy being particularly important to observe. Indeed, reports of sexual abuse may be lower in ethnic minority groups because disclosures significantly threaten family name and privacy. Thus, physical and sexual abuse are the two most common types of maltreatment that need proper and full understanding to avoid an institutional bias to over-report physical abuse, engage with families in a culturally sensitive manner with regards to both physical and sexual abuse, and protect children who have been physically and sexually abused.

Physical and sexual abuse get the most 'air time' because rates for these two types of harm are the highest across cultural groups. However, to ensure comprehensiveness and thereby look at all types of abuse and neglect, Chapter 4 also explores whether culture has anything to do with emotional abuse, inadequate supervision and neglect of basic needs across the rates of reporting found in the case files for the six cultural groups in Chapter 3, by triangulating qualitative interview data. In short, it is difficult to assess the role of culture in emotional abuse, and the criteria for neglect of basic needs seem to be relatively independent of culture. It is in the area of inadequate supervision that most reflects a risk for institutional bias and failure to sufficiently take culture into account. Reports of inadequate supervision could very well reflect culturally insensitive practice, allowing children who are not in fact being neglected into the child protection system and be vulnerable to its abuses. Extended family and communities have a greater role in parenting than in individualistic families and children are reared to be more responsible at younger ages, both of which could lead to false accusations of inadequate supervision by primary caregivers and the parentification of children.

Overall, the results show that of the six types of abuse and neglect studied, only physical abuse occurs for cultural reasons (physical discipline is culturally normative and acceptable), and for all types, especially physical abuse and inadequate supervision, child protection systems have a particular onus not to systematically commit institutional biases in their reporting. Perhaps most importantly, however, not all child protection matters for ethnic minorities are cultural in nature. Sometimes child protection matters have arisen because of some factor related to the *migration experience* such as intergenerational conflict or social isolation, which has impinged on the parent's capacity to care for their child well (discussed in Chapter 1). Sometimes child protection matters have arisen because the system has judged the family inaccurately by failing to look at culture appropriately or sufficiently, indicative of *institutional racism* (discussed in Chapter 2). But sometimes child protection matters have arisen because of some factor that could occur in any family regardless of their cultural background, described here as *generalist issues*.

Chapter 5 explores five such generalist issues – domestic violence, alcohol or drug issues, mental health issues in the carer, homelessness and poverty. Briefly, the case file data and qualitative interviews show that these issues occur for all families regardless of their cultural background but could be mistakenly attributed to culture for ethnic minorities. For the purposes of this book, culture for ethnic minorities is seen as synonymous with collectivism and unless the collectivist value for the family, and all related values such as harmony, cohesion and honour are directly involved, attributions to culture are inaccurate. In other words, poverty is not a cultural issue and domestic violence is not a cultural issue, but because ethnicity is so hard to ignore, caseworkers could falsely attribute such things to 'culture'. Migratory, generalist and institutional causes of entry into the child protection system are not cultural in nature (discussed more clearly in Chapter 10). If culture is repeatedly and falsely blamed as the primary cause for child maltreatment, then culture becomes stigmatised and pathologised, and enablers and perpetrators of other causes of abuse and neglect among ethnic minorities remain free from taking appropriate responsibility. Thus, Chapters 5 and 10 are critical for establishing what is and is not cultural in nature when ethnic minority children enter Western child protection systems.

Unlike Chapters 3 to 5, which focus on appropriately identifying risk factors to help make accurate attributions in child protection matters among ethnic minorities, Chapter 6 is about appropriately identifying protective factors which are also necessary for making accurate attributions in child protection matters among ethnic minorities. Family cohesion and willingness to engage in services despite cultural pressure to keep family matters private are perhaps the greatest cultural strengths, and attachment between parent and child is seen to be the most important non-cultural strength. Importantly, the expression of warmth through food rather than physical affection among collectivist families was noted and child protection workers are warned not to miss or dismiss this sign of attachment.

Chapters 7, 8 and 9 address discrete practice issues. Chapter 7 addresses how to work with interpreters effectively. The interview data in particular suggests that two types of training are necessary for improving practice in this area: training for interpreters so that they are aware of and sensitive to child protection matters, and training for caseworkers so they can competently facilitate a session. A range of relevant practice issues, such as the time load for caseworkers already time poor and working in unexpected and frequent crises, and finding a quality interpreter who will interpret verbatim, are also identified.

Chapter 8 looks at the costs and benefits of matching families to a caseworker of the same ethnic background. Overall, the results from the interviews show that this issue is best addressed on a case-by-case basis, as the pros and cons cannot be generalised for any family of ethnic minority background. As many as there are families who will feel comfort in having a shared ethnicity with a caseworker, in terms of language, culture and empathy, there will be as many who fear a matched caseworker, uncomfortable with the possibility that they will breach confidentiality and disclose their private family matters to others in the community and threaten their community standing.

Chapter 9 explores how children and families from different groups respond to being removed and placed in out-of-home care (OOHC). Overall, the results show that the trauma of removal is the same for families regardless of their cultural background, but that ethnic minority children would particularly benefit from matched placements to help preserve cultural identity. This is particularly true of long-term placements, but efforts to meet cultural needs should generally be considered in all cases. However, it may not be possible to meet the need for an ethnic-match because cultural stigmas make it difficult to recruit a large enough pool of ethnic minority foster carers. In light of this resource issue, it then becomes more important to consider the attachment of the child to the foster carer and the willingness of the foster carer to support the child's cultural needs. Care plans should also be detailed and tailored to the child's needs, having consulted with the family as a way of empowering and including them.

As stated earlier, Chapter 10 summarises the four main causes of entry for ethnic minorities into the child protection system: culture, migration-related stressors, generalist issues and institutional biases. In doing so, it is able to clearly differentiate cultural factors from other factors so that these other factors are not falsely seen as cultural ones. If this happens, culture becomes increasingly pathologised and at risk of being used as evidence to continue negatively stereotyping ethnic minority families.

By the time the reader has arrived at Chapter 11, typical child protection matters for ethnic minorities, being able to accurately assess their strengths and needs, working well with interpreters, considering whether to offer a matched caseworker and meeting the needs of removed ethnic minority children will have all been addressed. However, these issues all focus on the family and immediate responses to them when they enter the child protection system. Chapter 11 steps away from the most proximate unit to the topic of culture and child protection – the family itself – and moves into a wider, less proximate, layer that surrounds and influences that family. It starts by looking at barriers to cultural competency in child protection work, and argues that there are three levels that can inhibit practice at the focal point from being as well as it could be, delivering appropriate engagement with all ethnic minority families. The three levels are personal, organisational and institutional. Personal barriers may, for example, be racist attitudes held by caseworkers. Organisational barriers may include having management teams that do not reflect the local diversity, and institutional barriers may include insufficient allowance for the importance of culture in child safety assessment tools or poor data monitoring. A summary on how child protection workers, agencies and systems can be accountable for cultural competency has been provided.

In addition to summarising the key causes of entry into the child protection system and identifying barriers to cultural competency and how they could be addressed, the aim of Part III is to close the book, by wrapping up the issues raised and identifying directions for future research, practice and policy. In doing so, it provides a platform for expanding the research field, so as to acknowledge that the area of culture and child protection must remain open and ongoing, responsive to globalisation and its fluid and changing trends, with a value for changing and transformative practice.

A key feature of this book is that there are summaries of key points, recommendations for practice, and examples of good and poor practice from the case files and interviews throughout. Culture and child protection is a complex matter, and becomes increasingly complex the more attentive to nuance a caseworker is. Between- and within-group diversity can make the matter of culture in child protection so complex and overwhelming that it interferes with the necessity of taking it into account. In a time-poor service, marked by crisis and reactivity, the need for simple resources is also key to effective service delivery. To mitigate a risk to cultural competency, key points that can easily be considered during assessment and case management are needed, and the key points in this book aim to meet this need. Recommendations for practice help practitioners and policy makers see how best to implement the academic or theoretical literature and evidence into their work practice and act as brief resources that can be used by child protection workers, agencies and systems in Western countries to help improve culturally appropriate engagement with ethnic minority children and families. Examples of good and poor practice demonstrate when caseworkers and child protection systems are getting it right, providing cultural competency in their work, and when they are not, as lessons to be learned for the future. In other words, caseworkers can learn about the strategies that other caseworkers have used in ways that are either beneficial or not to ethnic minorities. Thus, the book is both scholarly and practical, providing evidence-based principles of best practice, rich with the inclusive and participatory voices of families and caseworkers, as well as user-friendly models and resources that take into account the crisis-driven, time-poor nature of the business of child protection work.

Like all people and cultural groups, the mainstream in Western countries fears a loss for their culture and its norms and values. This fear for the loss of one's 'way of life' repeatedly plays out as racism and discrimination in both everyday life and in historical events of big proportion (such as Nazi Germany against Jews, Blacks and immigrants, slavery of Africans in America, British colonial rule in India, apartheid in South Africa and the Stolen Generations in Australia (Sawrikar and Katz, 2010); the most current and topical being Islamophobia, and the mislabelling of asylum seekers as 'illegal immigrants' to justify detaining them and preventing their entry into Western countries like Australia). Such events across the historical and socio-political landscape keep 'White privilege' as a critical factor in the discourse on ethnic relations and racial equality. It highlights that the 'playing field' is not level and that a sociological framework is necessary when understanding ethnic minorities in Western countries. The fear among the mainstream in Western countries is understandable – it is human to want a place where one feels they belong and it is safe to be themselves. What it does not have in common with other cultural groups, however, is its power to protect its right to cultural preservation; minority groups face a much harder, difficult and uphill battle to preserve their same right. It is for this reason that the fear is unethical. In addition, change for the better can be excruciatingly slow, threatening to dampen the optimism and sense of empowerment of advocates for equality. Despite these challenges, every little effort counts. Thus, this book has been written in the spirit that if any change were to occur at all, voices that represent the rights of minority groups to hold on to and protect their (cultural) identity must at all times remain on the agenda of research, policy and practice.

Methodology
The study on which this book is based

This book does not claim to be exhaustive because it is difficult to offer such a thing on such a vast and complex topic, but great effort has been made to at least try. It is based on a large-scale three-year study, conducted as part of a Postdoctoral Fellowship between 2007 and 2010, on culturally appropriate service delivery with culturally and linguistically diverse (CALD) children and families in the New South Wales (NSW) child protection system in Australia. It was comprised of three stages: (i) a literature review, (ii) 120 case file reviews and (iii) 46 interviews. The study was co-funded by the state's child protection authority – the NSW Department of Family and Community Services (FaCS), then known as the Department of Community Services (DoCS) – and the Social Policy Research Centre (SPRC) at the University of New South Wales (UNSW). This chapter summarises the three stages of the study's methodology,[1] which were primarily qualitative but with some triangulation of quantitative methodologies.

Literature review

In the first stage of the study, academic literature and publicly available policy guidelines on child protection service delivery for ethnic minority groups were reviewed. The two main aims of the literature review were to identify the experiences, needs and challenges of ethnic minority children and families in the child protection system, as well as the experiences, needs and challenges of child protection staff working with them. Literature has been updated since 2008 when it was first conducted to ensure it is current at the time of writing.

Case file reviews

In the second stage of the study, 120 case files were randomly selected and reviewed from ten (nine urban, one regional) of FaCS' local Community Service Centres (CSCs); 20 per cultural group were explored: (i) Chinese [CHN], (ii) Lebanese [LEB], (iii) Pacific Islander – Samoan and Tongan [PAC], (iv) Vietnamese [VIE], (v) Aboriginal [ABR] and (vi) Anglo [ANG].

The first four of these are ethnic minority groups, selected because they have higher representations in the NSW child protection system compared to other ethnic minority groups (Sawrikar, 2009). Aboriginal[2] (or First Australians) and Anglo (or mainstream) families were also selected to make the point that culture is relevant for all families, not just those of ethnic minority background.

Other Western countries like the United States of America (USA), the United Kingdom (UK), Canada and New Zealand (NZ) have different demographic profiles to Australia. However, the experiences and processes that occur for ethnic minorities (and First Nation and mainstream people) are similar enough to yield this Australian data transferable to, and representative of, other comparable Western countries.

Case files were scoped for the following:

- Reported types of abuse and neglect;
- Reported risk factors of abuse and neglect;
- Reported strengths of children and families;
- Reported issues with the child protection system by families;
- Reported assistance provided to families;
- Examples of culturally appropriate and inappropriate practice;
- Examples of personal, organisational or institutional barriers to culturally appropriate practice.

The sample was representative of gender: 62/120 (51.7 per cent) were male. Children's ages ranged from 1–19 years,[3] with an average of 11.7 years (SD=3.8, n=120). The ages of the natural mother (NM; where reported) varied from 17–60 years, with an average of 38.3 years (SD=8.4, n=76), and the ages of the natural father (NF; where reported) varied from 27–67 years, with an average of 42.6 years (SD=9.4, n=39).

Country of birth was not stated in the case files of four Chinese, 13 Lebanese, seven Pacific Islander, ten Vietnamese, one Aboriginal and six Anglo children. The ethnicities of all 120 case files were only known because they had been manually verified by a caseworker before the reviews occurred at the CSC. For children where country of birth was recorded, most were born in Australia (n=57/79; 72.2 per cent) making them second generation.

Arabic was recorded as the primary language in only 13/20 (65 per cent) Lebanese case files. Vietnamese was recorded as the primary language in, again, only 13/20 (65 per cent) Vietnamese case files. The primary language of Samoan, Tongan or English was recorded in only 8/20 (40 per cent) Pacific Islander case files. Consistent record keeping was highest for the Chinese group, with 16/20 (80 per cent) case files having the primary language recorded as Cantonese, Mandarin, Chinese or English (n=2/16).

Religion was only recorded in 25/120 (20.8 per cent) case files. Of these, ten (8.3 per cent) were Christian (other than Catholic), eight (6.7 per cent) were Muslim, four were Catholic (3.3 per cent), two were Buddhist (1.7 per cent) and one had no religion (0.8 per cent).

While a total sample of 120 case files is large and robust for identifying relevant themes, the sample size of 20 per cultural group is not sufficient for conducting statistical analyses to test for cross-cultural differences. Thus, caution should be exercised when making inferences about each of the six *populations* explored. Having said that, the qualitative interviews (Stage 3) did reach thematic saturation, and triangulating three different sources of data (literature reviews, case file reviews and interviews) adds to the methodological strengths of this study. That is, a mixed methods approach to theory, data collection and data analysis all help improve the representativeness of a study's findings. Thus, the results overall are representative of ethnic minorities and child protection staff who work with them.

Qualitative interviews

The third stage of the study involved semi-structured interviews with 29 ethnic minority parents/guardians involved with the NSW child protection system and 17 NSW child protection staff.[4] Names of interviewees have not been provided to protect their anonymity and confidentiality.

The interview schedule aimed to be exhaustive and was informed by themes that emerged in the literature review and case file reviews. They explored:

- Norms, traditions, beliefs and practices that influence the way ethnic minority children are raised and family issues are addressed;
- Reasons underpinning the entry of ethnic minorities into the child protection system;
- Services provided to ethnic minorities;
- Perceived commonalities and differences in working with ethnic minority, Aboriginal and Anglo children and families;
- How caseworkers take into account different cultural contexts for children, while adhering to one Australian child protection law;
- Whether, and why, ethnic minorities and caseworkers prefer an ethnic-match;
- Examples of effective and ineffective practice with interpreters;
- Examples of culturally appropriate and inappropriate practice;
- The extent to which caseworkers perceive personal, organisational and/or institutional barriers impeding culturally appropriate service delivery for ethnic minorities;
- The extent to which the child protection system is perceived to sufficiently address the cultural needs of ethnic minorities;
- Suggestions for overcoming barriers to, and improving, the cultural appropriateness of child protection service delivery for ethnic minorities.

Of the 29 family participants [FAM_], ten were male (34.5 per cent), and interviewees varied in age from 22–67 years (M=42.2 yrs). Two were born in Australia, and 20 were Australian citizens, four were permanent residents, three were refugees, and one was a temporary resident.[5] The number of years lived in Australia varied from 1–45 years (M=18.9 yrs). Interviewees came from a diverse range of ethnic backgrounds (and spoke a range of languages) including from

Egypt, Iraq, Jordan, Lebanon, Turkey, Cambodia, Vietnam, the Philippines, Sudan, Burundi, Ethiopia, Ghana, Sierra Leone, Greece, Macedonia, Serbia, Maori, Samoa, Argentina and the Netherlands. Of those that completed the survey question on religion, ten were Christian (including Catholic, Pentecostal, Orthodox and Mormon), nine were Muslim, three were Buddhist and one identified as having no religion.

Of the 17 caseworkers, only two were male (12 per cent); however, this is consistent with the typically female-dominated social-workforce. Interviewees ranged in age from 23–59 years (M=33.9 yrs). The 13 non-English speaking background caseworkers [CW_NESB] originated from Afghanistan, Egypt, Lebanon, Burma, Laos, the Philippines, Vietnam, India, Uruguay and Ghana. Of these, four were born in Australia and so are second generation. There were also four Anglo caseworkers [CW_Anglo] and all were born in Australia. Three participants were case managers and the remaining 14 were caseworkers. The number of years working in their current role varied from one month to 14 years (M=3.8 yrs). A number of child protection staff made informal comments to the researcher in passing while based at their local CSC. Later, verbal consent to use their comments, without identifying them, was obtained from them [CW_ANON].

Collecting data from both service users and service providers is important for identifying their respective needs and experiences and where gaps in current service delivery may lie, and can be used as the basis for designing comprehensive recommendations for best practice and improve service in the future. The results of the interviews can also be compared and contrasted to the results of the literature and case file reviews, allowing triangulation of several data sources.

Notes

1   See Sawrikar (2009, 2010a, 2010b, 2010c) for the full original reports on which this book is based.
2   There are two distinct Indigenous groups in Australia: (i) Aboriginal and (ii) Torres Strait Islanders. In this study, only Aboriginal case files were selected to increase homogeneity and not merge their distinct cultural needs and experiences.
3   The age of the child, NM and NF was converted to 'years' by calculating the difference of 'DOB' (date of birth) from 31 December 2009. As a result of this computation, one child was recorded as older than 18 years.
4   As FaCS was known as DoCS at the time the interviews were conducted in 2009, all references to 'DoCS' from interviewees have not been changed to 'FaCS'.
5   Only 28 participants completed the question on citizenship in a short survey that followed the interview.

Part I

Setting the scene

1 Defining and understanding the client group

Who are ethnic minorities and what do they characteristically have in common?

Definitive characteristics of ethnic minorities

Getting the terminology right

Ethnic minorities go by many names in the literature. Sometimes they are referred to as the 'culturally and linguistically diverse' (CALD) and sometimes they are referred to as those of 'non-English speaking background' (NESB[1]). NESB was once the most common term used, but was superseded in the 1990s by CALD because NESB had come to have negative connotations; it was now code for 'the different other', and was limited in explaining the dimensions on which this group differed from the majority, which were not just along linguistic lines (Australian Bureau of Statistics; ABS, 2001).

At the time, CALD was seen as superior to NESB because it now drew attention to the fact that this group differs from the mainstream in both language *and* culture, and in celebrating the diversity *among* ethnic minorities, it was thought to be less subject to the criticism of referring to the non-mainstream. However, CALD and NESB are synonymous terms and so there was no escaping this issue: CALD still referred to people and groups that were not white and English speaking. If anything, it was worse than NESB, being covert or not transparent about the fact that it was actually differentiating groups that were culturally and linguistically *different* from the majority.

Moreover, CALD can be used not just in a categorical way to identify a sub-group of the population, but in a functional way to describe a (national) community as culturally and linguistically diverse, making the definition unstable and a term of convenience as to whom it wishes to include or exclude according to its end goal. In the main, it is used in a categorical way, thereby excluding the white English-speaking majority as if their culture and language were not sufficiently diverse to 'make the cut'.

For all these reasons, CALD is not the preferred term in this book and 'ethnic minority' is.[2] Ethnicity is a term that encompasses four key and relevant dimensions (O'Hagan, 1999) along which minorities typically face judgement for being different from the Anglo Saxon/Celtic, individualistic, English-speaking and/or Christian majority in Western countries:

- Race[3]
- Culture
- Language
- Religion.

That the terms NESB and CALD are synonymous indicates that language is a foremost demarcation of these groups from the English-speaking mainstream, and culture is indeed a critical variable that needed to be included, but in focusing on language and culture, CALD is not able to address racial barriers that ethnic minorities face. For example, migrants of German, Dutch or Irish ancestry differ from the mainstream in Western countries in language and culture but are not visibly different. They do not have brown skin, non-Caucasoid features or wear a hijab. Such visible markers of ethnicity mean that their barriers are sizeably less than their non-white counterparts. The term 'CALD' groups all of these together with the overall effect of masking the size of disadvantage for some ethnic minority groups compared to others (Sawrikar and Katz, 2009). By including race (and religion), which the term 'ethnicity' does, racial barriers – that is to say, racism and discrimination – are not at risk of being minimised.

Examples of good and poor practice 1.1 –
Language and cultural safety

We had a bit of problem [with DoCS]. Because we are Muslim, they were asking us how it was going to affect the child if we spoke [a] different language. [FAM_Maori]

[Anglo caseworker] told me 'speak Spanish. She has to learn Spanish. She can learn English when she start school'. That was something very nice he said. They want the kids to learn our culture. [FAM_Argentinian]

It's very interesting, as an Anglo person, coming into this organisation. It's been a very cultural experience. I've loved it. It's really exciting what you can learn. When we were training, they encouraged us, 'learn anything about the language of the people you deal with'. One time, it was an attempted murder situation on the [Vietnamese] mother and child. It was really serious at the hospital. I decided to say my [Vietnamese] 'goodbye'. I don't know what I said, but it brought tears to their eyes. They laughed and laughed! Culturally sensitive? I don't know?! [CW_Anglo]

It seems that human nature cannot help but see race, and has a strong propensity to attribute differences between groups to it, whether or not it is accurate. As an example, Indigenous children are substantially over-represented in the NSW child protection system at 25 per cent (Sawrikar, 2009), when their representation in the general population of NSW is only 2.2 per cent and in all of Australia only 2.5 per cent (ABS, 2006a, 2006b). This finding is not unique; 'the treatment of Indigenous children by the child welfare system reflects systematic racial bias right across the western world' (Barber *et al.*, 2000, p. 5).

What could possibly cause such gross over-representation if not, at some level, issues with the child protection system that assess these families and communities? No ethnic group is ten times more abusive than any other, for example. Perpetrators of child maltreatment come from 'all walks of life. Those who abuse children cannot be defined by race, class, religion or social status' (Sinclair, 1995, p. 160), and cultural norms make some things more or less acceptable in one group compared to another leading to over-representation in some forms of maltreatment among some ethnic groups, and some groups are at higher risk of maltreatment because of their higher exposure to risk factors like poverty (Bartholet, 2009), but this does not mean that Aboriginals are grossly abusive and neglectful of their children. To think this, is racist. It is a cognitively 'easy', and more importantly, risky, interpretation of the statistics. Instead, the large over-representation is indicative of injustice in the distribution of social, cultural, political and economic power (Fraser, 2005), and a historical effect where children removed and not parented by their own families are at risk of losing parenting skills across generations (see Chapter 2). To not be held accountable for such false inferences and attributions of maltreatment is to minimise discussions of racism. It is also a direct threat to the well-being of Aboriginal (and all) children.

Australian governments have also, more recently, intervened in these communities on the grounds that these statistics are evidence of high abuse. The 'Northern Territory (NT) Intervention' in 2007 was deemed necessary to protect Aboriginal children from the high sexual abuse and family violence in their communities. Yet, no such intervention has been carried out on Anglo families, and the data in this study – albeit small in sample size – preliminarily shows that the rate of reported sexual abuse and domestic violence is equally high in these two groups (see Chapters 4 and 5). Thus, the over-representation of Aboriginal children in the child protection system for sexual abuse (in particular) was seen by the government as evidence that 'ethnicity' was a predictor of sexual abuse.

Australia had clearly not learned from its mistakes of the past ('the Stolen Generations', see Chapter 2). That is, race (or culture or ethnicity, here acceptably synonymous) was seen to be the primary cause of sexual abuse, but of course, race was not openly named as the cause. Instead, culture was, perhaps even 'a culture of silence' (see Chapter 5). However, a culture of silence surrounds sexual abuse in all groups, so it was not really a non-racialised culture to which the abuse was being attributed; it was squarely a racialised culture that was being targeted, pathologising Aboriginal culture as if it were the root cause of the problem.

No doubt sexual abuse was occurring, and no doubt intervention was necessary to protect children in those communities, but if for this group then also for Anglos since rates seem equally high for both groups; child safety should be *equally* implemented across racial groups or it is simply racism. It is well established that sexual abuse is not condoned in any culture; it is not seen anywhere as normal, acceptable or of value. Thus, intervention along racial lines is racist (as the NT intervention was) and highlights how racism is at strong risk of being minimised if terminology does not allow for its inclusion and discussion. To prevent making such grave racist errors (over and over), it is critical that culture along racial/ethnic lines be defined if it is going to take any blame for abuse and neglect.

What is culture and where does collectivism fit?

Culture is a difficult word to define:

> Culture is that somewhat amorphous but quintessentially human orientation to life that allows us to interpret and give meaning to the social life around us. Culture is constantly changing defying easy definitions or the construction of a library-like catalogue of behaviors and values and instead demanding finely nuanced contextual understandings.
>
> (Korbin, 2008, p. 122)

Despite this difficulty, the word 'culture' at some *fundamental* level refers here to any time-honoured tradition passed from one generation to the next that is normal, acceptable and/or of value. Thus, there are many 'cultures'; there may be an 'Australian culture', an 'American culture' or an 'English culture', and there can also be a 'drinking culture', a 'stiff upper lip culture' and a 'tall poppy culture'.

Really, these cultures are just generalisations – stereotypes – that have emerged from normative trends and so have 'truth' embedded in them. Moreover, stereotypes are not inherently bad and should not be seen as 'a dirty word'. Stereotypes are adaptively useful and have evolved because they are cognitively efficient, buying us precious time when we think about our world in increasingly time-poor conditions. Stereotypes are only destructive when the beliefs that comprise them are untrue, negative and/or used to prejudge all members of a group. (Indeed, prejudice means to 'pre-judge', derived from the Latin *prae judicium*; Vaughan and Hogg, 2002.)

This means that if we are going to talk about 'racialised culture', or culture along racial/ethnic lines, then we are going to need stereotypes; we just need to be careful not to use wrong or negative ones or at all times. We need to use them with vigilance, ensuring that the beliefs comprising the stereotypes are accurate, do not perpetuate harm or disadvantage to groups and are questioned when applied to individuals. In the context of child protection, we also need to choose a stereotype that is relevant, appropriate and meaningful to a discussion on how ethnic minorities fare in Western child protection systems. To this end, the dichotomy between collectivism and individualism has been selected, consistent with other seminal researchers in the field (e.g. Maitra, 2005; Shalhoub-Kevorkian, 2005; Al-Krenawi and Graham, 2001; Hesketh *et al.*, 2000; Owusu-Bempah, 1999).

Overall, collectivism occurs in cultures that see the family to be the basic unit of society, and individualism occurs in cultures that see the individual to be the basic unit of society (Hofstede, 1980, 2001). More specifically, individualistic cultures value independence, autonomy, initiative and uniqueness, emphasise that individuals have the right and responsibility to look after themselves, stress horizontal relationships based on equality and tolerate deviations from the norm to a greater extent (Bond, 2002; Triandis, 1990). Thus, the concept of self is defined as separate and independent from the group, people define themselves in terms of individual attributes, the interests of the individual are given priority, the pursuit of fulfilment of individual goals is expected, behaviour is explained in terms of individual decisions and attributes, accumulation of individual wealth and possessions is the norm, and self-reliance, leadership, competitiveness, aggression and achievement are normal, rewarded and admired (Burton *et al.*, 2015).

Contrarily, collective cultures value social order, harmony, support and roles. In collective cultures the family provides security in exchange for loyalty and obedience, inequality (usually based on age and gender) is seen as appropriate and acceptable, and members tend to be more homogenous, as deviations from the norm are not tolerated as greatly (Bond, 2002; Triandis, 1990). Thus, the concept of self is defined only in relation to the group, people define themselves in terms of group attributes, the interests of the group are given priority, the interdependence and solidarity of people within the group are emphasised, the pursuit of group happiness and harmony are expected, behaviour is explained in terms of adherence to group norms, collective ownership of resources is the norm, and group conformity, obligation, sense of duty, collective responsibility and group/community-orientated achievement are normal, rewarded and admired (Burton *et al.*, 2015).

As they are stereotypes, it is important to point out that individuals are still of value in collective societies and family is still of value in individualistic societies. Thus, while there is truth to them and they are useful for making sense of our social world quickly, they should not be definitively relied on for individual children and families, from any cultural group:

> *There's this misconception that in an Anglo family, it's not strict. The children go off and do whatever they want. It's not the case. You have to take that into consideration and be careful. [CW_NESB]*

In fact, it is critical to remember that using this dichotomy reifies culture, treating it as if it were a 'fixed', monolithic or static entity (Korbin, 2002), rather than the highly nuanced and dynamic process of 'shifting interpretations and choices that individuals make from within their past and current experiences' (Maitra, 2005, p. 255). As Korbin (2002) notes, 'children are not passive recipients of socialisation into their culture. They shape and reinterpret it, and culture is experienced variably by different members of the group, and that interpretation and interaction are fluid' (p. 638).

Having said that, it is a human tendency to form stereotypes to help chunk the complexity of cultural issues, and this cognitive function cannot be avoided. Instead, it should be harnessed in a way that promotes cross-cultural equality. This can be achieved through the use of comprehensive and flexibly responsive schemas that contain key and accurate information about a culture's norms, values and traditions, as well as the pattern of variation around them, especially in relation to other variables such as gender, age, religion, generation, socio-economic status, education, employment, disability, sexuality (Babacan, 2006), neighbourhood (Roberts, 2008) and urbanicity (Kim *et al.*, 2011).

Hofstede has rated countries on their degree of individualism.[4] The data in Table 1.1 shows that the USA, the UK and Australia all rank highest and close to each other on individualism. They are also all Western countries. The implication of the data in this table is that all other countries, from which ethnic minorities in Western countries may originate, tend to be higher on collectivism.

In short, ethnic minorities are distinguished from their Anglo and Indigenous counterparts, refer to people and groups that originate from countries in which English is not the main language, may or may not be visibly different from the Anglo mainstream and tend to come from collective cultures. Refugees and asylum seekers usually fall under the term 'ethnic minority' too but have an additional set of niche experiences compared to other ethnic minorities who have chosen to migrate to Western countries (Williams, 2008; Lenette *et al.*, 2013; Hek, 2005; Davidson *et al.*, 2004; Taylor, 2004; Russell and White, 2001).

Table 1.1 Individualism (ID) scores by country

Country	ID	Country	ID	Country	ID
United States	91	Israel	54	Portugal	27
Australia	90	Spain	51	Tanzania	27
United Kingdom	89	India	48	Zambia	27
Netherlands	80	Argentina	46	Malaysia	26
New Zealand	79	Japan	46	Hong Kong	25
Italy	76	Iran	41	Chile	23
Belgium	75	Jamaica	39	China	20
Denmark	74	Brazil	38	Ghana	20
France	71	Egypt	38	Nigeria	20
Sweden	71	Iraq	38	Sierra Leone	20
Ireland	70	Kuwait	38	Singapore	20
Norway	69	Libya	38	Thailand	20
Switzerland	68	Saudi Arabia	38	El Salvador	19
Germany	67	United Arab Emirates	38	South Korea	18
South Africa	65	Turkey	37	Pakistan	14
Finland	63	Uruguay	36	Colombia	13
Poland	60	Greece	35	Venezuela	12
Czech Republic	58	Philippines	32	Panama	11
Austria	55	Mexico	30	Ecuador	8
Hungary	55	Kenya	27	Guatemala	6

Key points

- Ethnic minorities:
  - o   are also commonly referred to as the 'culturally and linguistically diverse' (CALD) and those of 'non-English speaking background' (NESB);
  - o   are distinguished from their Anglo and Indigenous counterparts;
  - o   primarily refer to people and groups that originate from countries in which English is not the main language;
  - o   usually also refer to people and groups that originate from collective societies;
  - o   usually include refugees and asylum seekers;
  - o   usually experience and perceive barriers to equal opportunity along racial, cultural, linguistic and/or religious lines.

Recommendations for practice

- ✓   Acknowledge that barriers to equal opportunity are not just along cultural and linguistic lines, but also racial and religious, and that as such 'ethnic minorities' is a better term than CALD or NESB, which both fail to allow for a discussion of racial and religious barriers.
- ✓   Language is critical for cultural identity, preservation and safety; its importance should not be under-estimated and should be encouraged at all times.

Cultural characteristics ethnic minorities typically have in common

Since ethnic minorities tend to originate from collective cultures, its characteristics help frame the client group. They also affect their needs and experiences once in the child protection system.

A value for strong family and community cohesion

Value for strong family and community cohesion (or 'togetherness') occurs in collectivist cultures because it protects the definitively important family unit. It is different to family cohesion as a result of economic dependency or need:

> *In Argentina, [children] stay with mother and father when they be 30, 40, 50 or all their life. We very, very close. Australian people not like that. They start to be like that now because [of] economical problems, but if not, they different on that. [FAM_Argentinian]*

However, it too varies among families of collectivist background:

> *Father explained his expectation of child at 16 years is that he should be out of home living independently and providing for himself. Mother does not agree with this. [CHN_case file]*

Family cohesion particularly affects the implementation of child-centred practice (see Chapter 2), and is a protective factor that should be fully considered in any 'strengths and needs' assessment of ethnic minorities (see Chapter 6).

Including extended family and community in child-rearing

It is normal in collectivist cultures to share child-rearing with extended family and community rather than leaving this task primarily to the nuclear family:

> *It's hard to raise kids in this country. It's easier and better in my country. Whatever my daughter do outside, no one cares. In my country, everyone cares. Like your neighbour watching your kids. Same, if I see any of my neighbours doing anything wrong, I jump [in] and say 'that's no good'. [FAM_Lebanese]*

Thus, families from collectivist cultures are used to expecting others in the community to have a role in the rearing of their children, that they play a role in others', and notice this as a differentiating experience between their country of origin and their new Western home country. This feature of collectivism has particular importance in the assessment of 'inadequate supervision' among ethnic minorities (see Chapter 4). It may also explain why ethnic minorities seem bewildered that Western countries have statutory child protection systems, with 'child protection' being seen as part of communities', not governments', role (see 'Lack of awareness of child protection systems' later in this chapter).

Since extended family and community play a significant role in the rearing of children in collectivist groups, it is worth consulting them when making risk of harm assessments and deciding the best interests of a child (O'Shaughnessy *et al.*, 2010). This practice is known as Family Decision-Making (FDM), a 'technique developed in New Zealand, applied through the medium of a Family Group Conference (FGC), that allows key decisions to be made by the family and friendship network regarding the welfare of one of their members, where the role of professionals is to provide information regarding assessments, supports, and resources' (Ban and Swain, 1994, p. 19).

**Examples of good practice 1.2 –
Family decision-making**

One of the most positive casework practices we have is consulting with other people and getting as much information as we can [to help] our decision-making. [CW_NESB]

We had a Tongan family – three children, domestic violence. We engaged the community – had a family conference with members of their family, extended family and church group. That worked well. [CW_NESB]

Practice issues that arise when using FDM with Aboriginal families (who are also strongly community-based) may also appear with ethnic minorities:

> *Difficulty with Indigenous families [is that] you don't know who you are really working with. You are trying to work with that parent [but] you've got [Aboriginal] professionals or family members who feel they have to have a say. We are not empowering the parents to make any decisions. Sometimes there are conflicts of interests – the parents decide one thing and a service or agency is advising another. [CW_NESB]*

Such challenges should not be used as evidence against the use of FDM; consulting with others may complicate matters, but it still helps caseworkers identify what is best for a child:

> *Child wants to live with mother but paternal grandmother fears that parents are not good because of drug problems and criminal history. [LEB_case file]*

Importantly, collaborating with people significant to a child is part of good practice for all groups, not just those with strong kinship values (Elliott *et al.*, 2001; Trotter and Sheehan, 2000).

Gendered child-rearing

In collectivist cultures, power differences between males and females are normal, acceptable, of value and overt; a striving toward more equally distributed power across gender is not as culturally normative as it is in individualistic cultures. Thus, child-rearing (and child maltreatment) may be gendered, with favouritism towards males:

> *She felt scared to disclose [the sexual assault] to her parents because she did not think they would believe her. There are privileges for males in the family and [Chinese] culture. [CHN_case file]*

However, child-rearing may also not favour males:

> *Children disclosed that the mother had hit them, mainly [male child]. "For some reason mum only hits me. Homework, I didn't bring it home, belting me with the wooden spoon. When my sister did it, she didn't do anything".* [LEB_case file]

The literature also reports that in collectivist and patriarchal societies, child-rearing is either harsher on boys because they will eventually have more power and responsibility for the collective, or harsher on girls to avoid them disgracing the family name. Both trends protect collective over individual needs:

> Chinese boys more than girls experienced severe violence at the hands of their parents (because) sons are expected to continue with the family line, take over the family business, and care for their aged parents. Thus parental expectations of and demands on sons are often much higher than daughters, and parents may turn to strict discipline to ensure their son's satisfactory performance at school as well as to train their filial behaviour at home.
>
> (So-Kum Tang, 1998, p. 388)

> The popular image of the Pacific region is of a peaceful paradise. However, in reality the Pacific is not idyllic for the girl child, who has a very low status in society, and is often subjected to various forms of violence, ranging from violent punishment at home and school, to domestic violence and sexual abuse and exploitation. This strict and sometimes violent treatment was intended to ensure the protection of a girl's reputation and a family's honour [and] prevent premarital pregnancy, which would disgrace a girl and her family.
>
> (Ali, 2006, pp. 3–6)

Gendered patterns of child-rearing are not just between parent and child but also between parents. In common with families of all cultural backgrounds, ethnic minority fathers may not partake in child-rearing to the same extent as mothers:

> *His wife dealt with children a lot more than him. He just didn't want to get involved.* [CHN_case file]

> *Due to limited opportunity for DoCS to engage with father, decision made for DoCS to close case.* [VIE_case file]

Several authors point to the difficulty of engaging fathers in child protection matters and call for their inclusion as much as possible (e.g. Zanoni *et al.*, 2014; Gordon *et al.*, 2012). Thus, gender is related to *culture* in the sense that patriarchal gender roles are patterned for all groups, and related to *collectivist culture* in the sense that the pattern is acceptable and overt.

A value for family name, family privacy and saving face

Among collectivistic cultures, where the family group is fundamentally important, 'anything a child does is seen as a reflection on the family name which must stay intact at all costs' (Elshaikh, 1996, cited in Giglio, 1997, p. 5). Babacan (2006) says, 'many CALD communities place a strong emphasis on morality within the family and consider maintenance of the family name, honour, shame and reputation within the community a high priority' (p. 6). Interviewees also said:

We teach children virginity and respect. [FAM_Lebanese]

We want to be proud of kids, 'my son is a doctor', 'my daughter is a professor at uni'. They love to spend money on their kids' education. [FAM_Lebanese]

Although he was born in Australia, want to raise child according to Vietnamese culture, so that later he can put himself in the right position in society, not like the Australians that use the words 'you' and 'I' without knowing which rank these people are interfacing. [So] when my kid see elderly people, they politely bow and greet them, not glance at them and then go away. [FAM_Vietnamese]

Disharmony or lack of cohesion within the family threatens family name and standing. For this reason, family problems are either not discussed or, more commonly, are only discussed within the nuclear or close extended family:

In our culture, we normally talk to relatives, not outsiders. [FAM_Sudanese]

In CALD families, the child has been brought up in a way where you don't talk about your family life outside. What happens in the home, stays in the home. [CW_NESB]

Importantly, the norm to keep family matters private is not exclusive to families from collective cultures, even though it is common:

I believe every family have their own secret. Something personal you cannot share. It has to stay and [be] solved inside the home. [FAM_Turkish]

It is also common in collective cultures not to talk to the wider community, as even this can threaten the family name:

We don't want other people to know our problems. It's for our own, you know? Because some [of] my people, once you ask for help or advice, they spread the whole story to other people. [FAM_Samoan]

If I live in America or England, I don't mind mixing with Ethiopian community. But here [Sydney] is a small community. They know who is who, what they do. When they meet in church or something, they talk about you and you become embarrassed. So you have to stay away from them. That doesn't help. [FAM_Ethiopian]

Thus, keeping matters private to protect the family name (even from extended community) is a key characteristic of collectivist families. This affects two main aspects of engagement with the child protection system – apparent prevalence of child maltreatment (see Chapter 3) and the tendency to seek assistance from external agencies (see Chapter 6), especially in regards to domestic violence (see Chapter 5), intergenerational conflict (see later in this chapter) and mental illness and other disabilities (see Chapter 5). The main implication for practice is the need to *clearly* assure ethnic minorities that all matters are kept confidential, except as required by law:

Paternal aunt wished to be anonymous. Mother is unaware reporter is giving a risk of harm notification. [LEB_case file]

Case Study 1.1 – The importance of confidentiality

Natural father (NF) not happy with service received. Dissatisfied with confidentiality (breach of trust). Said he wouldn't have said anything if he knew that info may be used in court. He made statement to get help [but] didn't receive the help he expected from caseworker (i.e. talk to NM). He trusted the Department even though he knew the Dept had a bad rep. He couldn't remember the casework manager telling him that info may be used in court [but he had]. Fears he is going to lose his family. [CHN_case file]

Religion

Religion is also a 'culture' that is important to consider when trying to understand the client group and how they fare in the child protection system. However, religion is different to collectivist culture. It is cultural in the sense that it is normative, acceptable and/or of value, and thus intrinsic to the group, but it is different to collectivist culture in which power across age and gender is overtly and hierarchically differentiated, and all norms and values ultimately aim to preserve the family unit.

Islam (and then Christianity) were most commonly noted by family interviewees as religions that influence their parenting values and practices, but more research is required on how religion is entwined with child protection issues:

Muslim families would be more difficult to work with than 'CALD families'. .
Then you not only take in cultural beliefs but religious beliefs [too].
[CW_Anglo]

It is not just important to understand how religious beliefs may impact on child maltreatment, but also how to improve engagement with families:

[In] the Australian culture, you can rock up to someone's house and start talking to them, [but] with different cultures, you have to be very careful in terms of how intrusive you are. In the Muslim religion, they would be very offended if a male picked up the phone and started having a conversation with his wife. If a male caseworker walks into someone's home and the female is on her own, that's also very offensive. [CW_NESB]

Research has shown that engaging with cultural awareness and sensitivity is a particularly crucial issue for Muslim families. Gray (2003) notes that 'Islam is perceived to be a challenge for Western society in general and for social and health services in particular' (p. 368), and Betts (2002) asks, 'can Muslim immigrants in Sydney be integrated in the same fashion as Orthodox Greeks or secular Chinese, or is the challenge qualitatively different?'. Importantly, Gray (2003) found that the centrality of Islam was played down (by white caseworkers) in an attempt to negate the religious beliefs of families and 'present everyone as the same' (p. 368), but this 'colour-blindness' affects the child's safety (see Chapter 2).

Key points

- Since ethnic minorities typically come from collective cultures, they have in common a value for strong family and community cohesion, the inclusion of extended family and community in child-rearing, gendered child-rearing and family functioning, and a value for family name and standing in the community and thus family privacy to save face.
- These collectivist cultural characteristics affect engagement with the child protection system.
- Collectivist and patriarchal culture is different to religious culture, and more research on how religion (especially Islam) affects child-rearing and family functioning is required.

Recommendations for practice

✓ Use cultural information to understand the client group, not to negatively stereotype them.
✓ Offer Family Group Conferencing (FGC).
✓ Involve fathers as much as possible.
✓ Strongly emphasise that all matters are kept confidential, except as required by law.

Non-cultural characteristics ethnic minorities typically have in common

In addition to collectivist characteristics, ethnic minorities also experience a cluster of issues that result from migration, affecting their needs and experiences both generally and in the child protection system. Importantly, these migration-related experiences (or acculturative factors) are different to cultural factors. Culture is intrinsic to a group, reflecting normative values brought with them. Acculturative factors are those borne of the migration experience and so are extrinsic to the group – they have occurred *because* of migration – but just because they cluster together for ethnic minorities, that does not mean they 'belong' to ethnic minorities.

It is for this reason that these issues are not exclusive to ethnic minorities. For example, socio-economic disadvantage tends to occur for ethnic minorities after migration but it also occurs for Anglo families, and racism and discrimination tend to occur for ethnic minorities after migration but they also occur for Indigenous families. It is also why not all ethnic minorities will experience all these issues; some groups will experience more acculturative stressors than others. Thus, it is simply that these non-cultural, migratory characteristics tend to cluster together for ethnic minorities.

It is important to distinguish cultural from acculturative factors when developing a broad framework that shapes the client group, because otherwise acculturative factors may be mislabelled as cultural ones (as if they belong to the group), and this risks that culture will be pathologised, or take the blame for being the main cause of entry of ethnic minorities into the child protection system. This risks feeding negative stereotypes about ethnic minorities.

Thus, 'the disorienting, stressful effects of migration' (Westby, 2007, p. 142) can impinge on the ability of parents to provide good care for their children and in turn 'increase the likelihood that children in immigrant families experience maltreatment' (Westby, 2007, p. 142). Having said that, migration-related stress interacts with cultural factors (e.g. keeping family matters private), creating complexity and, understandably, confusion about when and when not to attribute phenomena to culture. (See Chapter 10 for a delineation of cultural from non-cultural factors.)

Acculturative stress

For newly arrived families and groups, there is a period of steep adjustment and learning about the new country. These multiple and compounding factors can create a poor and difficult settlement period after arrival. However, stress that extends beyond the initial settlement period, affecting even established migrant groups, occurs as a result of continual pressure to 'fit in' with the mainstream.

This pressure is stressful; ethnic minorities consistently negotiate two contrasting cultural paradigms – individualism and collectivism – in their everyday life. These are also reactive to developmental, contextual, social and societal factors, such as their age, generation, ethnic composition of their social group and global trends in ethnic tensions (Sawrikar and Hunt, 2005).

Heuristically, this acculturative pressure can play out in four ways for either individuals or groups (Berry, 1980): (i) *integration*: high cultural preservation and high cultural adaptation; (ii) *assimilation*: low cultural preservation and high cultural adaptation; (iii) *withdrawal*: high cultural preservation and low cultural adaptation; and (iv) *marginalisation*: low cultural preservation and low cultural adaptation.

Thus, some families or groups may generally withdraw:

> *When Vietnamese migrate to Australia, they bring and strictly keep their culture. [FAM_Vietnamese]*

> *People come with a suitcase. That suitcase is not their clothes, but their traditional values. They are very guarded with them, very strict, thinking, 'I've got to keep this for my children'. [They] don't want to lose [their] identity. [CW_NESB]*

Others may generally assimilate:

> *My kids are born here so I raise them as normal Aussie people. I don't speak Cambodian [to them], I speak fully English. [FAM_Cambodian]*

> *I don't know [why you need to be] 'culturally sensitive' [in the child protection system]. You live in Australia, so you follow Australian rules. You bring up the child Australian, you do what Australians do. We're here now, so I don't bother about the Dutch culture. [FAM_Dutch]*

In short, acculturative stress is not exclusive to newly arrived migrants; it extends across generations. It affects sense of belonging and cultural identity, and perceptions and experiences of racism and discrimination, all together, affecting child-rearing, family functioning and engagement with the child protection system.

Displaced sense of belonging and cultural identity

As a result of being visibly different from the mainstream and/or being treated as different, ethnic minorities may question their sense of belonging and cultural identity. For example, Omar (2005) found that young Somalis, regardless of how long they had lived in Australia, felt distinct from other Australians because of their cultural practices and beliefs, language, race and physical appearance and skin colour, with religion and skin colour being the most significant of these.

Thus, a person who looks racially different may be treated as different even if they themselves 'feel' Australian. It may also be that non-visibly different minorities, such as Jews and/or white-skinned migrants, experience social exclusion that fuels a displaced sense of belonging or cultural identity and compromises mental health (Sawrikar and Hunt, 2005). The importance of preserving culture for sense of group belonging and cultural identity, as well as for cultural safety, is discussed in Chapter 6.

Perceived or experienced racism and discrimination

Ethnic minorities that are both visibly and non-visibly different may also have to cope with perceived or actual racism and discrimination. In the psychological literature, racism refers to the pre-judgement of an individual from a racial group based on a negative stereotype about that racial group (Allport, 1979). The sociological literature extends this by defining racism as a combination of prejudice and power; it is seen as 'a highly organised system of race-based group privilege that operates at every level of society and is held together by a sophisticated ideology of colour/race supremacy' (Cazanave and Maddern, 1999, p. 42).

Racism is also differentiated from institutional racism, in which:

> The (local) culture of an organisation – in its formal and informal rules, explicit and implicit protocols for workplace interaction and organisational memories – lead to a system of racialised oppression, the implication (being) that even if a white person does not discriminate individually, he or she benefits from white privilege based on group membership.
>
> (Feagin and McKinney, 2003, p. 19)

Discrimination is the enactment of racism and institutional racism. It may be exemplified by racialised taunting or scapegoating at the individual level and/or failure to actively commit to equal opportunity and multicultural policies at the institutional level (Chou and Choi, 2013).

Caseworkers and child protection systems should acknowledge that racism and discrimination are significant stressors for ethnic minorities. This can help avoid the trap of downplaying their effect because of the discomfort such topics can induce for either the caseworker (see Chapter 2) or the institution (see Chapter 11).

Socio-economic disadvantage

Ethnic minorities migrate to Western countries for socio-economic opportunities they do not have access to in their country of origin:

> *Parents moved to Australia to give children 'a better future'. [CHN_case file]*

However, upon migration, financial hardship is likely:

> *Parents always fighting about money. [VIE_case file]*

I've met heaps of parents, for example, they were teachers in their country, [but when] they came here, they found themselves [with] nothing. They have stress, heaps of problems, they don't know where to go, what to do. Even if they are educated, they have heaps of problems. [CW_NESB]

We don't get money from the government, and I'd like someone to support me financially because my children are at school. All the money we are paying for his studies [husband on student visa]. The children are feeling it. Often, they say they don't have enough in their lunchbox like all the other children and they feel they are different. And other activities at school, I cannot send them because I do not have money. [FAM_Jordanian]

Thus, financial issues borne of the migration experience include poverty and unemployment. (Also see Chapters 5 and 10.)

Loss of, lack of or isolation from extended family, social and community supports

Some ethnic minority families are satisfied with the amount of support they receive from family and friends and so do not feel socially isolated (see Chapter 6). However, social isolation can still commonly occur for ethnic minorities and in turn disrupt good family functioning, bringing them into the child protection system.

Much of the support of extended family and community they would typically rely on to help raise children is lost after migration. For example, Hartz (1995) speculates that the disproportionally high rates of abuse among Polynesian Americans might be related to the 'fragmentary assimilation into the larger culture' of the Polynesian extended family system and the loss of richly developed family and community networks caused by relocating from village life (cited in Pelczarski and Kemp, 2006, p. 11):

Family only recently having come to Australia from Samoa, were experiencing social and cultural isolation. [PAC_case file]

Mother's level of ability to meet the children's need of protection may be hindered by the lack of supports to assist with the large family rather than an issue of deliberate neglect. [PAC_case file]

Being in a new country, there's no extended families. That lack of support network around them, that isolation, is probably the biggest problem they've [CALD families] got. It's the biggest killer. Because of that, they then hit the drugs. With drugs comes the violence, with the violence comes the homelessness. It's [like] the isolation starts the cycle. It has taken me a long time to get to this realisation. [CW_Anglo]

Social isolation is not just due to lack of extended family and support networks; sometimes estranged relationships exacerbate feelings of social isolation:

> *Natural mother does not want to make friends as there is stigma in the community and she feels ashamed due to being divorced. [VIE_case file]*

> *Mum currently has no social supports and is socially isolated. Although she does have a family nearby, she does not feel emotionally connected to them. [CHN_case file]*

Importantly, child protection intervention can exacerbate social isolation for ethnic minorities. This is because 'the stress associated with coping with an allegation of abuse or neglect can fragment a family and isolate members from their community' (Westby, 2007, p. 141).

Intergenerational conflict

In the same way that 'traditional gender roles may become reversed, disrupting typical family dynamics' (Westby, 2007, p. 142), intergenerational tension between parents and children can also arise from acculturative stress within ethnic minority families. As Chand (2000) says, 'parents who feel their children may become influenced by the value system of the dominant culture may become stricter and more inflexible than usual' (p. 73):

> *Paternal grandparents complaining the subject child's (SC) clothing too seductive. Threatening to throw SC out of the home. [CHN_case file]*

> *A month ago, father disclosed an incident where child had ordered skin lotion on the internet. Arrived by courier. Delivery driver asked mother to open the package to make sure it was not damaged. When child found out mother opened it, child became very angry, screaming. She went to her father in the backyard. Father reported that he could not manage her level of distress and anger and hit her on the left arm with an open hand. [VIE_case file]*

> *Issues within family predominantly of a cultural nature. Child has been growing up in a Western world while his parents grew up in China. Since child has become an adolescent there have been recurring issues around food. Natural mother (NM) wants child to eat Chinese food when child wants to eat Western food. There have (also) been respect issues and NM did not deny she had hit child. It seems both parents only want the best for child, however cannot understand his adolescent behaviour. [CHN_case file]*

Importantly, intergenerational conflict has a normal developmental component to it, but for ethnic minorities there is an additional acculturative component:

Intergenerational conflict [for CALD families] – I don't know – is it a conflict of generation or culture? [CW_NESB]

Child is a normal 13 year old girl presenting with adolescent issues common at her age. Efforts to assert her own individuality. This is further accentuated by the cultural background of her carers which views assertiveness towards elders on the part of children as a sign of disrespect. [PAC_case file]

Thus, intergenerational conflict due to acculturation (not due to normal developmental processes) is a migration-related characteristic of ethnic minorities. However, this issue can interact with cultural factors, most especially the value for family privacy and protecting the family name, leading to tension for ethnic minority children experiencing maltreatment between two of their own conflicting needs – to seek help and protect the family name.

Children may want the assistance and representation of child protection services to protect themselves, but also fear that doing so will compromise their family's name and standing in the community. As a compromise, they may downplay the magnitude of maltreatment when caseworkers make risk assessments. As it is, child abuse has a 'secretive nature' (Bagshaw and Chung, 2001), regardless of the child's cultural background, but ethnic minority children 'may not openly express feelings about the abuse, in an effort to minimise intergenerational conflicts that might threaten ethnic or racial unity' (Markward *et al.*, 2000, p. 246):

Child told caller that she has a big secret but said the mother would kill her if she told the caller. Child is very aware of whom DoCS are. [VIE_case file]

Case Study 1.2 – Family privacy and intergenerational conflict due to acculturation

CW: *Do you know physical abuse is illegal? My job is to protect children.*

NF: *I am embarrassed and [feel] shame for this situation ... Children do not realise how much we love them, they do not recognise family values.*

Child [then] interrupted interview and admitted he was lying [about the physical abuse] because he was angry with his mother. Child recanted allegation. Concerns held this is rehearsed. [CHN_case file]

Low English proficiency

Low English proficiency may result after migration, and limit the capacity of ethnic minorities to integrate into the Western country and engage effectively with the child protection system:

> *Language is a barrier which may prevent mother seeking assistance. It makes it hard for her to access services for her and her children. [VIE_case file]*

Language issues were commonly found in the case files: 13/20 Vietnamese, 8/20 Chinese, 6/20 Lebanese and 2/20 Pacific Islander case files reported using an interpreter. The provision of an interpreter can assist in overcoming language barriers, but associated practice issues still need to be addressed (see Chapter 7).

The provision of translated documents can also assist in addressing language barriers, but its associated financial cost needs to be considered:

> *Dept of Immigration does not have translated copies of family violence provision in Mandarin. Referred me to naati.com.au.[5] Translate document cost approx. $300. [CHN_case file]*

> *The translation of documents [is] definitely a practical priority. [But] who pays the fee to have all the court documents translated, so that they have a fair understanding and don't have to rely on the five minutes they get with their solicitor? [CW_Anglo]*

Insufficient awareness of local services available

For a range of reasons, ethnic minorities tend to have low awareness of family and other support services available in their local community. One of the main reasons is cultural – the use of social services is uncommon in collectivist cultures because the trend is to rely more on family than the state in times of need or trouble (see Chapter 6).

Another reason may be past, fearful experiences with governments in the country of origin, which can cause them to withdraw generally after migration, and in turn perpetuate their lack of awareness of services:

> *[Some CALD families have a] fear of government services, especially from where they come from, [so] they have limited awareness of services [in Australia]. [CW_NESB]*

However, other non-cultural reasons also play a role. For example, a lack of translated and widely disseminated information about services, indicative of a systemic trend in which language diversity is not properly addressed, could account for low awareness of them. It may also be that ethnic minority families, like all groups, only become aware of services when there is a need for them. Thus, they are not actively seeking out information about them when family dysfunction is 'low-level' or emerging.

Fear of authorities

As one caseworker said:

> *[For] most of our clients, it's a shock having DoCS knock on the door, regardless of who you are or where you are from. [CW_NESB]*

However, fear of authorities – child protection, police, courts, taxation, immigration and housing departments – is generally heightened for ethnic minorities (Sawrikar and Katz, 2008):

> *Mother is terrified of authority. Reporter is concerned if DoCS or some other authority turn up to the house it will push her over the edge. [VIE_case file]*

Again, one reason may be the cultural need to protect the family name and keep matters private from authorities, and another may be negative experiences with authorities in the country of origin:

> *In particular, CALD groups have fear of authority. [CW_NESB]*

> *[To] a Vietnamese family who has come from a communist country, to say the police might become involved, is hugely scary for those people. [CW_Anglo]*

Fear of authorities may also be legitimate if there is illegal migration status and/or fear of deportation. As Giglio (1997) says, temporary residents may not report abuse or maltreatment for fear of non-receipt of citizenship:

> *Illegal citizenship status reported. [CHN_case file]*

> *Natural mother (NM) paranoid she will be returned to China. Mother and child on a temporary spouse visa. Dept of Immigration has a family violence provision – if there is abuse then Immigration won't send her back home – however there needs to be evidence of the abuse to support this. Mother and child are in fear that if they speak out about the issues, the relationship with the step-father will break down and they will be deported from Australia. [CHN_case file]*

Overall, Križ *et al.* (2012) report several fear factors when engaging with Western child protection systems – fear of deportation, fear of child protection workers as the people who remove children and fear of the child protection system as a potentially repressive government agency. These fears likely interact with a general lack of sense of entitlement common among ethnic minorities. For example, Križ and Skivenes (2011) report that 'caseworkers (in California) were of the opinion that minority families lack a sense of entitlement, whereas Whites, even if they live in poverty, have a sense of entitlement to prompt and fair treatment by child welfare workers and other professionals' (p. 1870). These authors ask a crucial question: do ethnic minorities make actual use of their citizenship? Thus, the pervasiveness of the fear of authorities among ethnic minorities is indirect evidence of their minority status, their lower social power.

Insufficient awareness of institutional systems, especially child protection

The trend among migrant groups is that they are generally not aware of how institutional systems, especially child protection, operate nor their roles. One reason is the sheer complexity of systems:

> *In Egypt, [the] law is easier than here. Here, too much stress. [FAM_Egyptian]*

> *Here [Australia], too much systems confuse people. When you drive a car and the window screen is cracked, that little crack, you keep leaving it there, cracks into a bigger one. If they have cracks back home, at least they're cracks in their own system. But here it's a crack in a foreign place. It is worse. We ask for a better life, but we can't deal with the complications in our new environment. [CW_NESB]*

However, ethnic minorities (both newly arrived and established) are generally not aware that the role of child protection agencies is to protect children who have rights, according to the United Nations Convention on the Rights of the Child (UN CRC). This is commonly due to child protection laws being either non-existent or not widely practised in their country of origin:

> *No DoCS in Vietnam. [FAM_Vietnamese]*

> *Natural father advised he had never heard of the Dept. [CHN_case file]*

> *Someone tell me, here government can take the kids, but in my country, never. [FAM_Lebanese]*

> *She clearly misunderstood the system, stating that she called the police because "in China police come to help with naughty children". [CHN_case file]*

> *CALD communities don't know what we do [or] what we are about. I'm from a non-English speaking background [and] I wouldn't have had a clue who DoCS was when I was a young kid. [CW_NESB]*

> *Child protection is underrepresented in some countries. They don't know, for example, [that] children have rights. And multicultural communities, even*

after some time, don't know about Australian rules and how they apply to them. [CW_NESB]

The strong pattern calls for the need for outreach programs to increase awareness of child protection systems in ethnic minority communities (see Chapter 11).

Key points

- Ethnic minorities tend to experience a cluster of issues that are each often mislabelled as cultural issues but are in fact issues due to migration (cultural issues are inherent to a group; migration-related issues are not inherent to a group but occur for a group).
- These migration-related characteristics can interact with cultural factors (especially keeping family matters private), disrupt good family functioning and affect engagement with the child protection system. They include (but are not limited to):
  - o   acculturative stress (for both newly emerging and established migrant groups);
  - o   displaced sense of belonging and cultural identity (especially for visibly different minorities);
  - o   perceived or experienced racism (personal or institutional) and discrimination;
  - o   socio-economic disadvantage;
  - o   loss of, lack of or isolation from extended family, social and community supports;
  - o   intergenerational conflict;
  - o   low English proficiency;
  - o   insufficient awareness of local services available (because of cultural trends to rely on family rather than external services, language barriers or perceived lack of necessity);
  - o   fear of authorities (which may or may not be legitimate, may be related to past experiences in the country of origin and is often strongly tied in with cultural factors of shame and minority status);
  - o   insufficient awareness of institutional systems such as child protection (because they are non-existent or not widely practised in their country of origin and/or because institutional systems are generally complex and overwhelming).

Recommendations for practice

- ✓   Consult with a 'multicultural caseworker' to help accurately separate cultural from acculturative causes of entry into the child protection system.

✓   To help address social isolation and low awareness of local services available, develop and translate pamphlets with definitions of child abuse and neglect, descriptions of institutional processes and procedures and options for addressing family dysfunction (e.g. local family and relationship services, parenting programs, playgroups, multicultural services, etc.).

Notes

1   'NESB' is defined statistically as a person who was born or who has at least one parent born in a country where English is not the main language spoken (ABS, 2007a).
2   CALD has only been used when there is direct reference to the study on which this book is based, as that project was funded under the title *'Culturally appropriate child protection service delivery for Culturally and Linguistically Diverse (CALD) children and families'*. Also, ethnic minority caseworker interviewees have been coded as [CW_NESB] in this book because it is a clearer/more self-explanatory shorthand than [CW_EM]; NESB is not seen to be problematic in the way CALD is – with connotations of exclusion to both minority and majority groups; it is simply seen as limited in thematic scope because it focuses only on language.
3   In this book, 'race' refers to phenotypic differences that carry 'social weight' (e.g. Asians having cosmetic surgery to their eyes, Africans straightening their hair and Indians lightening their skin colour, all to look more 'white'). It is not referring to 'race' as it is used in the genotypic-focused literature, which in fact demonstrates that differences are so small they nullify the term (Satzewich, 1998).
4   www.clearlycultural.com/geert-hofstede-cultural-dimensions/individualism/
5   National Accreditation Authority for Translators and Interpreters Ltd.

2 The theoretical backdrop

Why is it important to work effectively with ethnic minorities and across cultures in Western child protection systems?

Introduction: Culturally appropriate assessment tools and accuracy

There are so many reasons why it is important to work effectively with ethnic minorities, and with families across all cultures – mainstream and non-mainstream – in Western child protection systems (discussed in this chapter):

*   Ethnic minorities have less power (social, cultural, economic and political) than the mainstream and so struggle harder to preserve their right to be different in the way they parent and function as families.
*   Ethnic minorities are subject to child protection law that mostly reflects mainstream cultural norms of good parenting and family functioning, so deviations from those norms and claims of maltreatment are in turn ethnocentric.
*   The cultural needs of ethnic minorities are not addressed to the same extent as Indigenous families for whom cultural safety – protecting and preserving culture – is also important.
*   Ethnic minorities are represented in the child protection system roughly proportionate to their representation in the general community, but poor data collection masks this, making it seem they are less represented and used as evidence that the cultural needs of ethnic minorities can remain low in institutional priority.
*   Ethnic minorities are at risk of becoming over-represented in the child protection system when ethnocentric, rather than culturally appropriate assessment criteria, are used to judge whether maltreatment has occurred.
*   Culture is more at risk of taking the blame for over-representation in the child protection system than institutional racism (where organisational practices and policies preserve only the dominant culture). This has already occurred with Aboriginal children from and after the Stolen Generations who are over-represented in most Western child protection systems, as if the 'poor or primitive parenting' in that culture were the main cause of entry into the child protection system rather than assumptions of superiority by the 'white and civilised'.

- There are so many different ethnic minority groups that caseworkers cannot be expected to know all their different cultural norms; but this overwhelming complexity can then be used as grounds to continue using ethnocentric assessment tools.
- Caseworkers unfamiliar with the cultural norms of ethnic minorities may mislabel maltreatment as culturally acceptable (and therefore not harmful) behaviour, or mislabel culturally acceptable and non-harmful behaviour as maltreatment. The first risks a child's safety because maltreatment is missed, and the second risks a child's safety because children become open to abuses in the child protection system, such as families dealing with false allegations of abuse or neglect, the trauma of removal and/or abuses in the foster and other out-of-home care (OOHC) systems.
- State intervention can also further disempower families already disadvantaged and oppressed by their minority status.
- Ethnic minorities may defend maltreatment in the name of culture, and avoid developing insight into the harmful effects of maltreatment on children, if state intervention does not acknowledge their capacity to further disempower ethnic minority families or their need to engage with families in ways that respect their right to be different.
- Caseworkers who fear being seen or labelled as racist may exacerbate the risk of maltreatment being mislabelled as culturally acceptable and therefore not harmful, and thus fail to protect ethnic minority children.
- Some behaviours are both culturally acceptable and harmful, making culturally sensitive engagement even more critical as the vehicle to protecting children.
- Child-centred practice is difficult to implement with collectivist families because social power is overtly and normatively lower for children than older people.
- The strength of family cohesion as a protective factor could be overlooked if ethnocentric assessment tools are used to judge the strengths and needs of non-mainstream, collectivist, families.

Really, the list goes on.

- Not all causes of entry into the child protection system are cultural in nature for ethnic minorities, but their culture is at risk for taking the blame for these non-cultural (i.e. migratory and generalist) causes (discussed in Chapters 1 and 10).
- Low English proficiency and ineffective use of interpreters prevent ethnic minority families from being able to express themselves fully and therefore compromise the accuracy of caseworkers' assessments of maltreatment (discussed in Chapter 7).
- Lack of awareness of child protection issues, systems and their statutory power may lead to ethnic minority families disclosing more than their

Indigenous and Anglo counterparts and thereby becoming over-represented in the child protection system (discussed in Chapters 1 and 4).

However, to answer the question simply – and simplicity is welcome in such a complex matter – there are two main reasons why it is important to work effectively with ethnic minorities and across cultures in Western child protection systems. The first is that it is an issue of *child safety*, ensuring that children within a cultural group are safe from harm, and the second is that it is an issue of parity or *equity in child safety*, ensuring that children across cultural groups are equally safe from harm.

Further, these two things are related: the only way that all children can be equally safe from harm is through the accurate assessment of children at risk of harm. Accuracy 'hits two birds with one stone'. It protects not just one child in the best possible way, but all children in the best possible way and therefore to the same standard. If assessment of each child is driven first and foremost by the need for accuracy, then equity in child safety is also assured.

Accuracy, however, requires full and serious consideration of culture since culture, and its values and norms, are embedded in the way individuals, families and ethnic groups make sense of 'risk of harm', 'abuse' and 'neglect', and differentiate 'harmful' from 'not harmful' behaviours. As Gough and Lynch (2002) put it:

> Culture is perhaps the most basic issue for child abuse and child protection. It is the context in which children live and something to which they contribute. It is the backdrop against which all circumstances and events affecting children occur. It provides the basis for both our definitions of abuse and neglect and the responses we have developed to protect children and prevent abusing acts from occurring and recurring.
>
> (p. 341)

Thus, accurate assessment of risk of harm requires appropriate and sufficient consideration of culture and is the only way that all children in multicultural countries can be equally protected from harm, regardless of their cultural background. Actually, this fact is not difficult to appreciate, and child protection systems in Western countries go to great lengths to ensure that variables related to 'culture' like race, language and religion are embedded in legislation. What is difficult is putting it into practice, and equally for all groups. As Dutt and Phillips (2000, pp. 37–8) say, 'although professionals are aware that is essential to take account of race and culture, and to be culturally sensitive in their practice, they are often at a loss to translate this into practical terms' (cited in Chand and Thoburn, 2005, p. 169).

Working out when, how and to what extent culture should be considered in child protection matters is no easy task. There are so many factors that need to be identified and addressed when trying to 'get it right'. If they are not taken into account well – that is to say, in the right way and to the right extent – then a child's safety may be compromised, or the safety of children from one cultural group may be systematically more compromised than the safety of children from another cultural group. The first risk – to child safety – occurs if child protection practitioners and systems take a culturally relativist position towards the issue of culture and child protection, and the second risk – to equity in child safety across cultures – occurs if child protection practitioners and systems take a culturally absolutist position towards the issue.

Cultural absolutism – a risk of institutional racism

What is cultural absolutism?

The issue of how to address culture in child protection matters is evidently complex. For example, Harran (2002) reported that, 'social workers found it difficult to understand diversity and cultural difference and therefore understanding what is the norm and what is deviant becomes problematic. (They) were overwhelmed by the number of factors which appeared to be relevant to ethnic minorities and had difficulty in combining these factors in assessments' (p. 411).

Cultural competency (discussed in Chapter 11) also demands of caseworkers 'an understanding of the range of intra-cultural variability that arises along dimensions such as generation, acculturation, education, income, gender, age, temperament and past experience' (Korbin, 2008, p. 125), and because 'variability within groups often exceeds that between groups, and because populations continually adapt to changing circumstances, culture cannot be viewed as being uniformly distributed or having a uniform impact on all members' (Korbin, 2002, p. 638). All this complexity begs for simple, structured, decision-making guidelines. One way to create simplicity and deal with the difficulty of how to take culture into account is to reject the need to consider culture at all. This approach to child protection work in multicultural countries is known as 'cultural absolutism'.

Cultural absolutism is a theoretical attitude or stance towards the practice of child protection work in which culture and child maltreatment are seen as different and therefore separable things. The main implication of this is that culture does not need to be taken into account when deciding on the type and level of child maltreatment that may be occurring. In this way, it is able to 'offer' a standardised and colour-blind approach that equally protects all children regardless of their cultural background.

What is the problem with cultural absolutism?

The problem with cultural absolutism, as appealing as these offers may be *prima facie*, is that the standard has in fact emerged from, evolved across and become normed against culture. Sensically, that culture is the dominant group's culture: conceptualisations of child maltreatment are based on what is normal in the Anglo mainstream since they comprise the majority. However, as Western countries become increasingly multicultural, it becomes increasingly unacceptable to judge other families by a standard that is not applicable to them, and when it does occur it is known as institutional racism:

> Tools and instruments are used in child protection organisations in the belief that they are culturally neutral, universal and appropriate to all. This assumption fails to recognise that any child protection practice is closely related to the context and cultural environments within which it is developed. Given that tools are generally developed from research undertaken with Western, English-speaking people, they may not be applicable to other ethnic groups.
>
> (Connolly *et al.*, 2006, p. 47)

Thus, the institutional culture and processes of child protection systems in Western countries – a microcosm of society at large – cannot use one ideal of what constitutes maltreatment and then claim to protect all children from harm. This is ethnocentricism and serves to minimise the importance of culture for the child's safety, and 'cultural safety' (Papps and Ramsden, 1996) more generally – the need to protect and preserve the different cultures of different groups. In short, culture is a variable of extreme importance in child protection work in multicultural countries because it helps guard against institutional racism – when only the dominant culture is protected by policies and practices that essentially judge different others as 'not normal'. It cannot be dismissed on the grounds that it is complex.

Chand (2000) suggests that it is the inability or unwillingness of practitioners to distinguish 'abuse' from 'cultural practice' which lies at the core of an ethnocentric approach. More broadly, 'ethnocentrism reflects a belief that one's own cultural beliefs and practices are not only preferable but also superior to all others' (Korbin, 2008, p. 3). As a result, failure to challenge the ethnocentric family norm, and design and implement policies and practices that are sensitive to cultural variation in conceptualisations of the family, creates a situation where appropriate service delivery for ethnic minority families becomes predicated on assimilation – a (covert or overt) forced imposition of suppressing cultural ideologies of 'the family' among ethnic minority groups that are not in line with the cultural values and ideologies of the mainstream.

Several authors note this. For example, Barn (2007) says, 'a cultural deficit perspective makes it a mission to alter and correct "pathological" cultural learnings to ensure their alignment with the supposed but elusive "norm", leading to what may be described as speedy and unnecessary over-interventions in the lives of ethnic minority children and families' (p. 5). Similarly, Korbin (2008) says, 'to overcome an ethnocentric approach to protecting children requires an orientation towards cultural difference rather than deficiency. A deficiency approach is ethnocentric while a difference approach allows a more circumspect and contextual perspective without compromising child wellbeing' (p. 124).

Markward *et al.* (2000) say:

> It is common practice to assume that similarities exist across individuals and groups in order to produce some kind of consensus for research ideology and diagnostic purposes. Unfortunately, such generalisations often lead to negative stereotyping that is predicated on racial and ethnic prejudice rather than substantive comprehension of cultural nuances. The attempt to establish behavioural norms for all minority cultures, based on the assimilation myth of a 'melting pot' disallows new learning and social evolution and/or reorganisation in favour of mislabelling diversity as individual defect or deficiency.
>
> (p. 238)

Maitra (2005) also points out that:

> It is important to distinguish between 'needs' and 'ideals'. Child protection (should) aim to ensure the prevention of significant harm, rather than ensure optimal/ideal development ... Further, it is crucial not to refer to 'needs' as universal, and failure to comply with preventative programs as 'neglect', when in fact they more indicate the 'ideals' of the writer.
>
> (p. 256)

In short, an absolutist approach to child protection work risks mislabelling a culturally normative and non-harmful behaviour as abusive or neglectful, simply because it is different to (an irrelevant) norm. At worst, it can result in the removal of a child otherwise safe from significant risk of harm, causing more trauma to the child and their family had authorities not intervened, and overriding their very function – to protect children from harm. The child would also be open to other forms of harm inflicted by the child protection system, such as possible maltreatment in the foster or other out-of-home care (OOHC) systems. Applying one cultural yardstick for assessing what is 'harmful' can systematically bias ethnic minorities in their entry into the child protection system.

The Stolen Generations: a historical example of cultural absolutism

Australia has already made the grave and horrid mistake of cultural absolutism. Overt policies of assimilation in the past (the 'White Australia Policy') imposed cultural absolutism on Aboriginal children and families and from 1910–1970, somewhere between 1 in 10 and 1 in 3 Indigenous children were forcibly removed from their families and communities to be 'saved' from themselves and 'civilised' by superior white families and institutions (Burton *et al.*, 2015). These children and families of 'the Stolen Generations' are subjects of ethnocentric policies of assimilation, supposedly bettering 'different' families but instead inflicting intergenerational trauma and harm at the hands of institutional processes and policies not, in fact, designed to help children and families:

*With Indigenous families, this is their original country. [But] when you
haven't been parented, you can't parent. Your ability to form and maintain
relationships [is affected]. The degree of brokenness is so severe.
[CW_Anglo]*

Indigenous children the world over have been oppressed and disempowered by
supremist ideologies of Western colonisers including in the USA (Lu *et al.*, 2004)
and Canada (Trocmé *et al.*, 2004). 'The existing child protection system; the laws,
values and assumptions of the "dominant culture" are embedded in the mire of
failure of successive governments to provide culturally sensitive programs'.[1]
'Social workers (in the UK) have underestimated or misunderstood the ability of
black families to raise their children and have inappropriately intervened in the
family process' (Chand, 2000, p. 70).

Positively, there has been acknowledgement of the limitations of cultural
absolutism and ethnocentrism, and there is now a far greater body of evidence and
interest in the preservation of culture for First Nation people around the world.
Unfortunately, this same acknowledgement does not extend to ethnic minorities.
While they have not suffered structured policies of assimilation to the same extent,
the cultural loss for children would be the same; what is at stake is the same. As
Babacan (2006) notes, 'recent government initiatives have attempted to address
cultural deficiencies in Indigenous service provision, however the CALD
population has largely gone unnoticed' (p. 11). Legislative policies and procedures
are in place for meeting the cultural needs of Indigenous children in Australia, but
such policies are not in place for minority ethnic groups (Kaur, 2007):

*From what I've seen, Aboriginal clients have a better chance of receiving
better treatment than CALD groups. I've got a [CALD] family that needs
financial assistance. The paper has been lying there for about four weeks. At
the same time, the Aboriginal cases get processed much [more] rapidly.
They're just trying to make sure they respond to these things quickly, so that
no one can use that against them. I cannot comprehend this unevenness.
[CW_NESB]*

*The practice [is] a lot more effective with Aboriginal families. There's
Aboriginal consultation, secondary Aboriginal caseworkers, a big unwritten
rule about Aboriginal families having access to Aboriginal supports. Because
there's so many different ethnic groups under 'CALD' you can't possibly
meet all those [needs]. [So] the practice in terms of consultation, although
it's not up there, is much better for Indigenous families than it is for CALD
families. The policies are there. They are worked into the legislation in terms
of kinship carers. CALD families don't have [that]. They don't address it as
part of routine practice because no one pushes it. In our care plans, it will ask
you things about Aboriginal or Torres Strait Islander [but] it doesn't ask you
anything about any other culture. We've got checklists produced by HO
[Head Office], [but] I would dare say, most people here have never seen [or]*

> *used them. When there is a checklist that comes out for an Indigenous family, it is made compulsory, people have to do it. So yeah, the Indigenous structures are much better than the CALD ones. They both need a lot of work [but] it won't get fixed for a long time. I suspect [it will] take a while for the organisation practice and mindset to change. [CW_NESB]*

(The need for mandatory consultation for ethnic minority client families is discussed in Chapter 11.)

Slow research and poor data collection with ethnic minorities risks repeating history's mistakes

The capacity to fail to protect the 'cultural safety' of ethnic minorities grows if it is left unchecked and unaccounted for. That is, research and knowledge-building in cultural capacity, with commensurate funding, are essential to good practice and performance measurement (Tilbury, 2006). As Petrova (2001) puts it, 'how can a budget aimed at compensating structural disadvantages be developed if the number of persons in the disadvantaged category is unknown?' (cited in Krizsán, 2001, p. 9).

Research on culturally appropriate engagement with ethnic minorities has been repeatedly, and for a long time, noted in the literature as slow to develop, lagging in responsiveness to changing population demographics (Bromfield and Arney, 2008; Cashmore *et al.*, 2006; Miller and Cross, 2006; Thoburn *et al.*, 2005; Korbin, 2002; Burke and Paxman, 2008; Pinderhughes, 1991). As Welbourne (2002) puts it, 'culturally competent practice (in the UK) with a strong commitment to the principles of empowerment and of countering oppression and discrimination is so fundamental in child protection interventions that one might expect a well developed literature on the subject ... In fact the literature is surprisingly small' (p. 345).

A more aggressive accusation of why research on cultural issues has been slow to get proper attention is institutional racism: not acting quickly in ways that could promote equity perpetuates and maintains disadvantage for some groups. A more benign explanation for why the design and delivery of culturally responsive models for ethnic minorities has been overlooked is because of their apparent under-representation in the child protection system. Researchers may omit comment or analysis of issues around ethnicity because the small sample sizes compromise the reliability of data (Chand and Thoburn, 2006):

> *The service provided to CALD families is a more 'as-you-go' type of response. [CW_NESB]*

> *[There are] no specific programs for CALD families that I know [of], but this CSC doesn't have the CALD numbers to justify this. [CW_NESB]*

Despite the development of policies and sincere attempts by agencies to meet best practice principles and accreditation requirements around respect for cultural identity, there is a degree of ad-hoc response and inadequate preparation of staff and carers for the complexities involved in supporting children and young people from CALD backgrounds. As long as numbers of CALD clients in general and of particular cultural background clients remain small, it is difficult for agencies to develop the skills of staff and to have resources fully developed to assist when such clients are referred or placed. The lack of 'critical mass' of CALD children in the care of any single agency make such evaluation and planning a low priority given the demands of service delivery.

(Chuan and Flynn, 2006, p. 23)

However, apparent under-representation can be attributed to poor data collection. For example, it only became mandatory to collect data on variables related to a child's ethnicity such as the child's or parents' country of birth, the main language spoken at home other than English or the child's cultural ancestry/identity in the NSW child protection system in Australia in 2009.

Since such data had not been routinely collected until then, representation of ethnic minority children was inaccurate and under-estimated. According to FaCS' Multicultural Services Unit (MSU), the database indicated that only 4 per cent of the total population of children in the NSW child protection system were of children that spoke a language other than English at home, but an internal audit revealed that it was closer to 15 per cent and the figure became nearly 20 per cent after adjusting for the over-representation of Indigenous children in the child protection system[2] (Sawrikar, 2009). This is nearly on par with the representation of non-English speaking background (NESB) groups in Australia's general population at 24 per cent (ABS, 2007a)[3]. The international literature points to similar trends. In King County, Washington, for example, Hackett and Cahn (2004) found that 76 per cent of records in the database listed race as 'unknown'.

It is also important to note that ethnic minorities span a diverse range of languages, cultures, races and religions, and grouping them together falsely homogenises their needs; Fontes (2005) calls it 'ethnic lumping'. It fails to acknowledge diversity (opposite to the main aim of cultural research), but it also makes it difficult to identify groups with the *most* need because the overall size of disadvantage or inequity is masked by those groups who experience fewer barriers (Sawrikar and Katz, 2009). Unfortunately, such issues can be difficult to avoid. As much as possible, they should at least be acknowledged.

In short, data collection is necessary to ensure that the cultural needs of ethnic minorities are not minimised or that child protection systems absolve their responsibility to provide a culturally competent service because of apparent low representation. (See also Chapter 11 on mandatory data collection.) Arguably, the over-representation of Indigenous Australians necessitates caseworkers to be aware of and sensitive to their needs. This need can be avoided for ethnic minorities with good data collection and research on how to prevent over-representation of ethnic minorities due to culturally insensitive practices and policies. Allowing history to repeat its mistakes of the past, through avoidance of the importance of culture or minimising the damage that could be caused for ethnic minorities, is unacceptable. The consequences could be across generations, entrenching and making irretractable over-representation:

> *Talking generically, a lot of the families we deal with have been through the child protection system when they were younger. This is why they are lacking those parenting skills, because they were never parented with those skills. Parenting skills are a learned behaviour. If you don't see it when you were a child, how do you know what's the right thing to do when you have children? That's inter-generational. I have a 13 year old and I can bet my life on it, we are going to repeat the cycle with her. We are going to remove her children – she doesn't even have children at the moment – [but] given that I know what the 13 years of her life have been like ... Her mother was removed, she's been removed, and there's been no insight anywhere along the line. [CW_Anglo]*

Entrenching the cycle of (over-)representation in the child protection system, at some point, will lead to families taking some of the blame for not having good parenting skills; later attributions of cause of entry into the child protection system become difficult to disentangle – is it due to culturally insensitive policies or the family or both? Research on culturally appropriate practice and the development of best practice models with ethnic minorities must play serious 'catch up' and get the proper attention it deserves, before children become over-represented in the child protection system at least due to institutional biases. As Boushel (2000) says, 'we need to be committed to documenting the lived experiences of minority populations to help redress racism' (p. 85).

Key points

- To be able to work effectively with ethnic minorities and across all cultural groups in Western, multicultural child protection systems, accuracy in risk of harm assessments is required. In turn, accuracy requires appropriate ('how') and sufficient ('how much') consideration of culture, and ensures that each child is as safe from harm as possible and therefore that all children are as safe from harm as possible to the same extent; that is, accuracy ensures both child safety and equity in child safety.
- In multicultural countries, a pressure arises to adopt one standard to help simplify the task of making accurate risk of harm assessments across many different cultures.

- In Western countries, that one standard is often falsely seen as 'universal' and independent of cultural factors ('cultural absolutism') but in fact tends to reflect mainstream norms. This is because culture is the 'substrate' that gives rise to norms on parenting, risk, harm, abuse and neglect and so is never irrelevant. However, because their norms are more easily accessible, by virtue of being the majority culture, ethnic minorities can be judged against norms irrelevant to them and which (overtly or covertly) expect them to assimilate.
- Ethnocentricism – where one group's culture is used as a reference point by which to judge others because of an assumption of their superiority – has already occurred with First Nation people worldwide with devastating consequences to children and families, including intergenerational brokenness and over-representation of Indigenous children in Western child protection systems.
- Poor data collection on variables related to culture facilitates institutional racism because it indicates that the needs and experiences of ethnic minorities are low in institutional priority, and perpetuates the use of ethnocentric organisational and institutional policies and practices that preserve one group's culture but not others'. It also leads to a false under-representation of ethnic minorities in the child protection system, which can then be used as evidence to continue keeping it low in priority.

Recommendations for practice

✓ Acknowledge that assessment tools of abuse and neglect are never independent of culture; thus, culturally appropriate/relevant/applicable norms for each child need to be considered for accurate assessments of maltreatment.

✓ Data collection on variables related to culture (e.g. ethnicity, ancestry, country of birth, languages spoken other than English, English proficiency, etc.) should be mandatory to improve the accountability and performance measurement of the child protection system.

Cultural relativism – a risk to child safety

What is cultural relativism?

The opposing stance towards child protection work in culturally diverse communities – cultural relativism – acknowledges that culturally applicable norms for each child need to be considered for accurate assessments of maltreatment. It takes responsibility for voicing the importance of culture in child protection matters. It does not avoid an onus to act. It is not afraid of the complexity associated with culture, the effort required or the ensuing subjectivity across caseworkers in its implementation. Its main purpose is to address the ethnocentric pitfall of cultural absolutism. It also values self-determination and equality. In the words of Pedersen (1989), 'cultural dimensions do matter when examining the ethics of autonomy … "Do not onto others as you would have them do onto you. Their tastes may be different"' (p. 651, cited in Yick, 2007, p. 283):

> *Culture should be a massive part of your case plan no matter what background a family is from. A service might be appropriate for an Anglo family and completely wrong for a Greek family. [CW_Anglo]*

> *It's really important a caseworker understand culture, so they can understand the whole case. They shouldn't treat people the same way, because every culture is different. Something 'normal' for some cultures, something abnormal for other cultures. [FAM_Turkish]*

> *Most people work with them [CALD families] the same. The problem is they are different. For example, it's quite unlikely you are going to find drug and alcohol issues with an African family. With Anglo families, that's on the forefront. We will get, say an Asian family [with] serious physical abuse, but it's all based around education, so the abuse isn't based on inadequate parenting capacity, it's based on the fact that education is one of the paramount things of that culture. With an Anglo family you wouldn't see that. If you are [only] looking at, 'this is the law, you're not allowed to do this', [that's an issue]. A lot of the time, knowledge of the cultural background will explain why the primary reported issue is there. Everything you do as a caseworker with an Anglo family in comparison to a CALD family should be quite different, but it's not. [CW_NESB]*

Korbin (2008) states that 'cultural relativism is the belief that every culture must be viewed in its own right as equal to all others, and that culturally sanctioned behaviours cannot be judged by the standards of another culture' (p. 123). This approach emphasises that 'most behaviour has to be seen in context before it can be thought of as maltreatment' (Chand, 2000, pp. 70–1).

Thus, cultural relativism acknowledges that culture and abuse are embedded and therefore cannot be separated, thereby offering to take culture into account seriously. It starts by putting the family and their culturally relevant context at the forefront of decision-making and using this as the basis for whether maltreatment has occurred. In the words of Korbin (2008), assessments of abuse and neglect are based on whether the behaviour is considered 'proscribed – acts that even within the cultural context are prohibited by the culture' (p. 124). This approach to the diagnosis of harmful behaviour avoids ethnocentric impositions of judgement, and therefore the mistake of mislabelling a culturally normal and not harmful behaviour as maltreatment.

Case Study 2.1 – Focusing on child safety without considering culture

When I read the report [that] the woman was going to chuck her baby because she was fed up, I automatically thought, 'CP' instead of thinking about the culture. You just have that crisis sort of mind-frame. We totally ignored the fact that this woman is from another culture. She was brought up in a home where she was very well off, everything [was] done for her, they had slaves in the house. It was totally shocking to her. She was like, 'look, I'm a bit frustrated, but I don't physically want to throw my baby. I love my baby. I don't understand'. We were thinking, 'why doesn't she seek help?' We didn't understand. It's important first to look at who the person is, and why they might be saying or doing what they are doing, because at the end of the day, the answer was quite simple. She just needed someone to reassure her a bit that it's alright to seek help. Caseworkers need to take into consideration cultural differences before they react. [CW_NESB]

One of the main problems with cultural relativism: behaviours that are culturally acceptable and harmful

As useful as cultural relativism is for more accurately identifying whether maltreatment has occurred, one of the main problems with it is that some behaviours are not proscribed by the cultural group but they are still harmful. Child-rearing practices may be legitimised in that culture and have the intent to be helpful but are in fact harmful (Chan *et al.*, 2002).

The most extreme example of this cited in the literature is female genital mutilation (FGM) or female cutting. As Koramoa *et al.* (2002) put it, 'the problem with traditional cultural practices such as FGM is that it both enhances a child's cultural identity and causes them harm' (cited in Gough and Lynch, 2002, p. 342). Westby (2007) says, 'a relativist approach allows abuse such as FGM because it is perceived as a responsible act by the parents that ensures their daughter's place in society, but no practice that is harmful to a child should be condoned in the name of culture or tradition' (pp. 141–4). Another more common example of behaviour being both harmful and culturally acceptable is the use of physical discipline among many ethnic minority groups (see Chapter 4).

Thus, the problem with an exclusively relativist approach is that it permits harmful practices to children that are conducted because they nevertheless serve important cultural functions. Cultural relativism is also consistent with an assumption that 'parents act in the best interest of children' (Chan *et al.*, 2002, p. 365), and reflects 'a rule of optimism – the belief that parental/family love can override different and/or punitive manifestations of child discipline' (Chand,

2000, cited in Barn, 2007, p. 5); but all the while, there is a compromise to the child's welfare and 'respect for cultural diversity' allows it. Indeed, Sale (2006) points out 'there is a lot of language bandied around about "respect" and "respecting others" but social care has not worked out how to respect a culture while acknowledging its limits' (p. 28):

> *Cultural norms about what we think are acceptable and what they think are acceptable comes as a challenge. [CW_Anglo]*

Example of good practice 2.1 –
Normalising cultural differences in child protection work

Sometimes the line is very blurry between what we see as child abuse and what CALD families see as everyday living and culturally appropriate. It's just talking with them and breaking it down, saying, 'look, I understand that it's part of your culture, but you need to understand that from our perspective, it is a child protection concern'. Don't play it up and don't say, 'you are a bad parent'. Just explain that it is a difference that we deal with all the time. [CW_Anglo]

The importance of engaging effectively

When behaviours are both harmful and promote cultural functions, engagement that is respectful *and* protective of children becomes critical:

> *Engagement is so important because without that, you cannot move into more difficult areas later. CALD families are respectful, if you give them culture. [CW_NESB]*

Example of poor practice 2.2 –
Lack of cultural sensitivity and ineffective engagement

There are caseworkers who have underlining racism issues, which you can't sift out as much as you'd want to. [For example] some caseworkers just don't care about cultural differences, 'this is it, this is our bottom line, these are our CP concerns, I don't care what your reasons are, this is what is going to happen'. You are going to get off to a bad start with families straight away. [CW_Anglo]

Koramoa *et al.* (2002) identify a continuum of child-rearing practices. They note that if behaviour is deemed *beneficial*, then caseworkers should preserve and promote it (e.g. breastfeeding, infant massage); if behaviour is deemed *neutral*, then it should be understood and respected (e.g. toilet training at 1 year); if behaviour is deemed *potentially harmful*, then both caseworkers and families should be educated about the possible harm (e.g. circumcision); and finally, if behaviour is deemed *harmful*, then it should be prevented (e.g. chilli in vagina, FGM, honour killings, forced marriage and extreme neglect). The useful and concrete examples were offered by Raman and Hodes (2012).

Example of good practice 2.3 – Not mistaking 'neutral' as 'potentially harmful' behaviour

I had a family who were Fijian Indian and their son had drug issues. We removed his baby. I had been to see the grandparents and the place was clean, tidy. They cook outside, however. I didn't have a problem with that. The manager said that's not acceptable. 'They're going to keep the child outside while they cook, or the child's going to be inside?' To take into consideration, culturally, [that] that's how they cook, all their stuff is outside, they had set it up, there's nothing wrong with that. [But] they had a problem with that. I fought and eventually the child got placed there. [CW_Anglo]

Two risk factors: misplaced defensiveness in families and fear of being seen as racist among caseworkers

Culturally appropriate engagement is also critical because ethnic minorities may feel further disempowered by government intervention on top of their minority status, in turn, causing them to cite the cultural normality of their behaviour as acceptable grounds to continue the harmful behaviour. As others have said, 'cultural identity is so central to group membership and thus personal identity that any suggestion of the negative effects or inappropriateness of a (cultural) practice is likely to be sensitive, particularly if pressure for change comes from outside the culture condoning the practice' (Koramoa *et al.*, 2002, cited in Gough and Lynch, 2002, p. 342), and 'applying Western values to collectivistic groups, mainly in relation to obligatory reporting and involvement of the official system, causes additional trauma and social harm to abused children, which may prevent victims of abuse and caregivers from recognising or acknowledging child (sexual) abuse in the same way as in Western countries' (Shalhoub-Kevorkian, 2005, p. 1265).

It is possible that defensiveness in ethnic minorities is heightened from a fear of being culturally misunderstood. However, such defensiveness is only likely to cause the family to misplace their focus on their perception or experience of feeling pressured to conform to the practices and values of another, dominant, culture, instead of on the harm their parenting practice is causing their children.

The risk of 'denial of abuse' (Webb *et al.*, 2002) among ethnic minorities may also be exacerbated by white caseworkers who fear being labelled racist, ignorant or culturally unaware (Westby, 2007; Sale, 2006; Maitra, 2005; Williams and Soydan, 2005). As Brophy *et al.* (2005) put it, 'a (potentially or actually harmful) practice or behaviour cannot be accepted as cultural simply because the parent says so. However, because culture is so politically charged, workers may hesitate to challenge parental or caregiver explanations' (cited in Korbin, 2008, p. 9). Barn (2007) also says, 'the "race awareness" training industry, perhaps contributed to white social workers feeling guilty, deskilled and powerless, and may have resulted in the kind of professionals who sought refuge in "cultural relativity" models of thinking' (p. 3):

> *You get it all the time – [accused] as being racist, at having no idea what it would be like – especially with blonde hair. [CW_Anglo]*

> *Absolutely [feared being thought of as racist]. I don't think you cannot. I'm a white young female walking into a family that I don't know a lot about. It could be viewed as racist. How you get past that, I don't know. The approach that often works [is], 'I don't know about you, your family, your culture, tell me about it.' [CW_Anglo]*

Overall, fears of being labelled racist or culturally unaware can impact the caseworkers' ability to manage ethnic minorities in denial of child maltreatment. These families may instead displace responsibility for maltreatment on a structurally racist system. Maitra (2005) describes this in the following way:

Parents who have a genuine emotional investment in their children may nevertheless make one-off (or more) errors of judgment. Afraid (of state authority), ashamed (at having allowed or caused harm to children they care about), humiliated (at being investigated), angry (at their beliefs and practices being questioned), and buoyed by the often ambiguous benefits of ethnic community lobbies urging 'empowerment', BME (black and minority ethnic) parents (in the UK) may often appear aggressive, threatening, non-compliant, untruthful, and more interested in questioning professional authority than in considering how they may be better parents. Skilled risk assessment must allow for these tensions and yet identify those parents who have little genuine commitment to their children and may be attempting to cover up serious maltreatment. Errors have serious negative consequences and not only because of failure to identify risk. In addition to the dangers of separating children from essentially loving parents, embattled relationships between ethnic communities and services increase the risk of social exclusion of these children from mainstream society.

(p. 256)

The other main problem with cultural relativism: failing to protect a maltreated child

At the very least, 'conflicts over child rearing practices in an ethnic community that would be considered child abuse in the broader community reinforce the need for discussion about what constitutes child abuse' (Giglio, 1997, p. 6). However, it also highlights the second main issue to child safety with cultural relativism: the sheer complexity of needing to be aware of all different cultural norms.

In arguing that cultures are so different from one another that they cannot and should not be compared, child protection systems are left with no cross-cultural consensus on what abuse and neglect are. This makes it hard for caseworkers from a background different to their client families to identify when some children are being abused or neglected, and in turn, possibly missing the maltreatment and failing to protect them. As Westby (2007) says, 'the UN Convention does not spell out just what is considered to be abuse, (and) cross cultural differences in childcare standards complicate the issue of determining just what should be considered abuse with a particular child' (p. 142).

Cultural relativism values the uniqueness of cultures to the point of removing all yardsticks, and this is challenging to good practice in multicultural countries. That there is no structured and agreed-upon definition of what constitutes 'abuse' (Clark, 1995) is problematic in multicultural countries, and attempts to empiricise and structure definitions of abuse and neglect (e.g. objectively determining 'significant' risk of harm) or family dysfunction (e.g. number of standard drinks consumed per month to substantiate alcohol abuse) make sense and are helpful during decision-making.

However, ultimately, all decisions in child protection work – not just those that relate to culture – rest on the subjective and interpretive professional judgement of caseworkers and case managers. As Harris and Hackett (2008) say, 'child welfare decision-making is never free of subjective bias. Caseworkers rely on intuition, experience and interview engagement to assess child safety, and decisions that permanently affect a child or family's fate are made on a daily basis by individual case workers, attorneys, service providers or judges' (p. 203). Similarly, Gillingham (2006) says that the process of risk assessment is itself not without its flaws, as it is not an exact science and requires a level of informed and interpretative 'art'. Munro (1996) further argues that initial assessments and professional judgements should be open to revision as a sign of good practice to 'overcome hasty or intuitive judgments that may be informed by a caseworker's own values and stereotypes' (cited in Harran, 2002, p. 412):

> *Legislation and policy guide you so far. Ultimately your professional judgement is what forms your views. Whilst you have one family you take one course of action with, there may be something that impacts this with another family. There's no hard and fast rule about how you address risk. Whilst there's definitions about what risk looks like, ultimately it's about the impact on the child and there's going to be different impacts for different families. [CW_Anglo]*

Thus, subjectivity is not actually problematic, and in fact is seen as essential and crucial to good practice, as each case is individual and individual analysis is the most appropriate form of intervention and aid. In the context of culture and child protection, valuing the subjectivity of decision-making means accepting the complexity and recognising the limits of using objective measures of abuse.

A threat to cultural relativism: providing only universal services

The two main pitfalls of cultural relativism are that (i) children who are being maltreated may also be gaining other cultural identity benefits and that is challenging to address effectively (i.e. respectfully and protectively), and that (ii) children who are being maltreated may fail to be detected because there are so many norms caseworkers would need to be aware of. Despite these problems, cultural relativism is still important because it avoids the use of a standard, ethnocentric approach to the diagnosis of maltreatment, keeping culture at the forefront of decision-making. It also highlights the importance of cultural sensitivity for effective engagement with families with lower socio-cultural power than the mainstream. One of the greatest threats to the importance of cultural relativism is the provision of *only* universal services.

Access to, and use of, universal services by ethnic minorities is critical for promoting equity; it indicates that families are treated in the same way when they should be. Positively, the case file reviews showed that ethnic minority, Aboriginal and Anglo families generally receive the same kinds of services. The most common were financial assistance and referrals:

- *Financial assistance* (e.g. camps for children, sport and recreation centres, short-term accommodation, vacation care, cost of computer, cost of moving furniture into storage, cost of car, rental assistance, groceries, sporting equipment, childcare, taxi vouchers to support services and school shoes).
- *Referrals* (e.g. anger management programs, mental health counselling, drug and alcohol counselling, domestic violence counselling, relationship counselling, bereavement counselling, school counsellors, sexual assault services, parenting skills training courses such as Triple P, early intervention programs, programs for fathers, addressing challenging behaviours in children, conflict resolution and assertiveness skills, women's housing group, and regular home visits from NGOs).

Universal services are also important because not all issues for ethnic minorities are cultural in nature. Thus, while culture is important, it should not be looked at to the exclusion of other factors.

However, the additional provision of culturally *appropriate* services is also important for ethnic minorities. Specialised, culture-specific services enhance engagement, and thus promote fairness and equity in the full use of services. As Westby (2007) puts it, 'harm can occur from inappropriate referrals and

---

**Example of good practice 2.4 –
Holistic and individualised approach to child welfare**

It doesn't matter who you are working with, you need to take into consideration not only their culture, but their situation. Like a Samoan mum who was hit when she was a child, and has come over here. It's a new country, you can't expect them to know the ins and outs of our laws and policies. Even their education levels play a part. They could be normal functioning people [and] a neighbour got pissy and made a report. Mental illness, drug abuse, the list could go on forever. That's why we have to come from a holistic approach. [CW_Anglo]

---

interventions by ill-informed ethnocentric professionals, which can lead to distrust, non-compliance and avoidance of services that would benefit the children and family' (p. 141).

Specialised services for Indigenous families already routinely occur; in nearly all 20 Aboriginal case files, referrals were made to Aboriginal support services (e.g. legal, educational, cultural pride, etc.). In comparison, only 19 ethno-specific referrals were made across the 80 ethnic minority case files (e.g. Vietnamese Women's Support group, Australian Chinese Cultural Association's Family Support Program, TransCultural Mental Health Service, Our Lady of Lebanon counselling for sexual assault, etc.).

Low referrals to culturally appropriate services may occur for two reasons. The first is that caseworkers may perceive the provision of such specialist services, for groups where culture is important, as a risk to (cross-cultural) equity:

> *[CALD families] should receive the same services provided to every other client. Our services shouldn't be, 'we're going to provide this to you and not to someone else', because that goes against our code of conduct and legislation, of DoCS' vision [for] fairness [and] equity. [CW_Anglo]*

However, interpreters are only provided to families who need it, so the fact that it is not provided to all families is not seen to compromise service equity. In this case, the specialised service, provided only to families who need them, makes sense – they are responsive to the needs of a family and cultural group, and in turn enhance accuracy in risk of harm assessments to be on par with other groups:

> *[We] use interpreters. That's the only main thing that's different [between cultural groups]. [CW_Anglo]*

Such an example makes common sense and generally does not generate emotive responses, because the language needs of an ethnic minority group are relatively easier to meet than their cultural needs and are an obvious barrier to equity.

Cultural differences, on the other hand, are more complex to identify, and more importantly, require institutional and systemic recognition and acknowledgement of differences in socio-cultural power between the mainstream and other minority cultures struggling to preserve their identity and way of life, under the weight of the dominant group's efforts to preserve their identity and way of life.

Some time ago now, O'Hagan (1999) said that 'culture is very often ignored, misunderstood, misinterpreted and/or intentionally downgraded, and that preoccupation with culture is criticised (because) there is insufficient recognition of the importance of culture in identity construction' (p. 278). Arguably, this has changed since the 9/11 bombings and all terrorist activity since, with Western countries becoming increasingly aware of and driven by a need to preserve a safe and free way of life. In other words, the importance of identity may have become stronger in recent times because it has now gone under actual threat.

However, the preservation of identity has been a core issue for ethnic minorities for much longer because it is threatened to be lost to the majority as soon as migration occurs. Ethnic minorities may, to some extent, accept there will be loss of some of their culture of origin, even embrace the opportunity to change and grow in a new culture, but in the end, discover that it is not humanly possible to (pretend to) be someone you are not. Identity is so core to the human experience that assimilation, and blending into one melting pot, is not possible. Visible differences in race and socio-economic differences in power vow to keep a sad fact – that not all people are treated equally or have equal opportunity.

Low referrals to culturally appropriate services may also be because caseworkers perceive their provision as a threat to child safety, as if the two were definitively at odds with each other:

> *The difficulty in the Department is with Indigenous cultures. It's so predominant over other cultures. We have every possible support you could imagine for Indigenous people. You tread so carefully. You have to have specific cultural consultations. Part of the Act is specifically around that culture, and that culture almost overrides child protection matters. Sometimes it's so blown out of context, and that's such a difficult thing to say, because I appreciate the utter sensitivity of how bad we have done, but the pendulum has swung so far the other way that we need to be careful that we are balancing that as well. [CW_Anglo]*

While caseworkers acknowledge that the 'line' between culture and abuse is subjective, some more than others see the need to consider culture as crucial to ensuring child safety, and others take a more 'bottom line' approach, citing that even though culture matters, it ultimately matters less than child safety. Really, there is no clear-cut 'rule of thumb' to help caseworkers differentiate between culture and abuse, especially since it may not even be appropriate to do so; culture and abuse are each themselves difficult to describe and categorise, and may be embedded within each other rather than being separable. This creates the subjective complexity that can drive caseworkers towards the 'absolutist' end of the pendulum.

However, the principles of universality and absolutism do not work for different children and families. They fail to tailor service to the different needs of different groups. Access to universal services is certainly one important way of demonstrating equity, but it is actually the provision of appropriate services rather than the provision of similar services that is the real measure of equity in service delivery. Walker (2002) also argues for 'equivalence in standards rather than exactly the same service being provided for all' (p. 384).

Thus, the provision of universal services does not replace the need for routine referrals to culturally appropriate services for ethnic minorities; this is when families should not be treated the same. Access and usage of service should not be seen as synonymous; just because a service is clearly acceptable to the majority does not mean it will be appropriate for everyone. Any attempt to reduce inequalities must acknowledge that this will not be achieved by simply providing more of what is accessible to the majority. Nutbeam (presentation to National Children's Taskforce, October 2002) has likened this approach to the English habit of saying the same thing again but louder to those who do not understand our language (cited in Gough and Lynch, 2002, p. 343).

Providing an interpreter is also insufficient for promoting equity, and should not be the only difference in service between groups. Cultural issues for ethnic minorities are not synonymous with, or reducible to, their language needs, and so offering to provide an interpreter forms but one part of good and culturally appropriate practice.

In short, similar service provision is an easy way of operationalising 'cross-cultural equity' but in fact it simply demonstrates a 'colour-blind' and therefore culturally absolutist (or 'one-size-fits-all') bias. The provision of culturally appropriate services is a better litmus test of whether there is equity in service provision; and knowing when and how to tailor services to meet the unique needs of an individual family or a cultural group is important for maintaining equity in the protection of all children. Culturally appropriate services protect cultural safety and therefore child safety, and cultural relativism promotes this. In the words of Humphreys (1999), 'white children may be often experiencing a second class service, (but) the service extended to Asian children (in the UK) can really be rated only as third class when, for a range of reasons, attention is not given to meeting their identity needs' (cited in Chand, 2000, p. 69).

'It is difficult for professionals to report abuse with immigrant families because there is a delicate balance to tread between being culturally sensitive, treating everybody equally, denying differing needs or believing in cultural deficits and accepting or applying a lower standard' (Westby, 2007, p. 146). To ensure cultural safety is not inappropriately separated from child safety, that cultural needs are not emphasised over other needs and that cultural identity needs are not reduced to language issues, several principles of good practice are required, of which one is equal access to universal services combined with routine referrals to culturally appropriate ones. Both are necessary indicators of parity in service delivery.

Key points

- Cultural relativism is a theoretical position towards the issue of culture and child protection, opposing cultural absolutism. It acknowledges that risk of harm assessments must consider culturally applicable norms to help them be more accurate; that is, to examine whether behaviour is seen as 'proscribed' or unacceptable to that cultural group first. In doing so, it treats each culture as equal in value and right to be, and avoids ethnocentric judgements that carry assumptions of superiority.
- One main problem with cultural relativism is that some behaviours are acceptable, normal and/or of value to a cultural group but are also harmful to children (e.g. female genital mutilation (FGM) and excessive physical discipline).
  - No practice harmful to children should be permitted in the name of culture.
  - Parents should be educated on the harmful effects of their practice, in a respectful way that does not further disempower ethnic minorities by state intervention.
  - If they are not engaged respectfully they may defensively displace attention onto their feelings of disempowerment rather than onto the harmful effects of their behaviour and on developing insight.
  - White caseworkers fearful of being labelled culturally ignorant or racist may struggle with managing ethnic minorities' 'denial of abuse'.
- Another key problem with cultural relativism is that needing to be aware of so many different cultural norms complicates the risk of harm assessment process. In not having some cross-cultural consensus on what abuse and neglect look like, some maltreated children could be missed and therefore failed to be protected.
  - This complication is not evidence for a culturally absolutist approach to child welfare in culturally diverse communities.
  - Instead, subjectivity in assessments needs to not just be accepted, but also valued as the means for providing a tailored intervention that meets the unique needs of each family.
  - In turn, it provides equity in the protection of all children regardless of their cultural background, because it takes a holistic approach that neither overstates nor overlooks the role of culture.
  - By corollary, the provision of universal services is not a sufficient sign of cross-cultural equity; it is a sign of a one-size-fits-all bias. *Access* to universal services should be equal, but the provision of culturally *appropriate* services is also required to improve cross-cultural equity.
  - The provision of an interpreter is not sufficient for meeting the cultural needs of ethnic minorities.

Recommendations for practice

✓ Do not downplay or fear discussions on culture or racism; acknowledging these can aid in developing an appropriate intervention with the family, and avoids implicitly condoning denial of maltreatment in their home.

Comparing and resolving 'cultural absolutism' versus 'cultural relativism'

Quick summary

It is important that 'culture is not mistaken for maltreatment and maltreatment is not mistaken for culture' (Korbin, 2008, p. 123). If caseworkers misattribute non-harmful parenting behaviours to abuse or neglect among different cultural groups, then it may indicate either a lack of cultural knowledge and sensitivity or institutional racism, both of which can cause disruption and trauma to the child and family through their unnecessary or avoidable intervention. On the flipside, if caseworkers prioritise culture over child safety, they risk contributing further harm to the child for failing to appropriately intervene. The first scenario results in 'false positives' or the over-identification of maltreatment in ethnic minority children, and the latter results in 'false negatives' (Maitra, 2005), or the under-identification of maltreatment. Both consequences fail to meet the needs of ethnic minority children and protect them from harm equally. Table 2.1 summarises these issues.

Table 2.1 Summary of the advantages and disadvantages of cultural absolutism and cultural relativism

	Cultural absolutism	*Cultural relativism*
Advantages	Offers a 'standardised' assessment of maltreatment regardless of a child's cultural background, and cross-cultural benchmarks are important in multicultural societies as is the need for an easy-to-use assessment tool that all caseworkers can implement.	Offers a culturally sensitive assessment of maltreatment, using culturally appropriate norms as the benchmark/threshold for differentiating harmful and non-harmful behaviour. In this way, accuracy in assessment is enhanced; ethnic minority children are less likely to be incorrectly judged as maltreated.

Table 2.1 continued

	Cultural absolutism	Cultural relativism
Disadvantages	The 'standard' assessment actually reflects mainstream cultural norms and so an ethnic minority child may be incorrectly judged as maltreated. Children, families and ethnic minority groups then become vulnerable to abuses in the child protection system. These can include (further) disempowerment from state intervention/removal, subjection to other culturally insensitive practices and policies or child maltreatment (e.g. emotional abuse) in the foster and other out-of-home care (OOHC) systems.	Caseworkers from cultural groups different to their client families may fail to detect maltreatment because they are not aware of culturally appropriate norms in different groups. If there are too many different norms to take into account, the process of assessment becomes complicated, which is also a risk to children. Behaviours may be both culturally acceptable/valuable and harmful, rendering culture an insufficient reason to be complicit with or condoning of child maltreatment. Denial of abuse among ethnic minority families and fear of being seen as racist by caseworkers both exacerbate the disadvantages of cultural relativism.

Which one is worse?

The risks of cultural absolutism and cultural relativism are equally problematic in terms of protection of children. However, their occurrence is currently not even. Understandably, child protection systems work off the principle that 'it is better to be safe than sorry', but as a result, it falls towards culturally absolutist practice, seeing that 'over-policing' families – removing children, leaving children vulnerable to the (emotional and other) abuses of the foster and other OOHC systems and introducing children to a culturally insensitive system – is better than leaving children with harmful parents. The liability to the system is not worth it to them. As Munro (2010) puts it, 'professional practice is being excessively controlled and proceduralised' (p. 1135), and 'in a defensive culture, the protection of the agency can dominate the protection of children' (Munro, 2004, p. 880):

> *Child indicated that DoCS is overdoing it. They are caring parents and not just because of the Dept's involvement. [CHN_case file]*

> *DoCS just want to cover their ass. They don't want to take any risk and so they record everything down as abuse. They used to have far more contact with services before they would remove. Now they just remove for everything. And just for two or three weeks. In that time, parents can kill themselves cos they think 'I've lost my child'. [CW_ANON]*

When I said to get my child back so that he can have breastfeeding, my culture was not respected. In our culture, when a lady gave birth she has to breastfeed. That's normally what we know, rather than artificial milk. I haven't asked anything apart from that. They are dealing with their rules. I ask that and no one accepted. They [caseworkers] scared themself not to do something else, not to do your request, when your request [is] out of line. [FAM_Sudanese]

Before they take the children from parents, they have to be very, very sure, they doing the right thing. Because if not, they completely ruin family, and doing the wrong thing. The first time I knew DoCS exist, was when they took my granddaughter. I was very angry with them. Oh my god, I hate them so much, because I can't understand how they can take children like that. But after, you see things, like the father kill the child, things like that, and I say, 'ok, somebody have to protect them, sometimes the parents doing the wrong thing. [Then] I said 'no, they're doing their job. And I think they're doing a good job'. But before they take the baby, they have to make sure they doing the right thing. [FAM_Argentinian]

Case Study 2.2 – Entrenched institutional fear

We're such a powerful agency. People are scared of us. They don't talk to us. [They] think that what we think is absolute. You don't want to remove children, you've got to work with the family, [but] in reality, you don't. All our work is based on legislation, [it's] very strict. This is the ugliest job I have ever had. We have to cover our butt – let's remove first, protect the child from risk. We have to be more relaxed about child protection. I know that some parents deserve to have their children taken away, [but] we have to not jump to the conclusion that 'children need child protection, children's rights'. Involve in the extreme cases [only]. We don't say, '[if] you place this child in foster care, they might abuse the shit out of this child'. You hate your job because you have to remove children, you don't have time for an extreme case load, and you've got this very unhealthy work culture [where] you don't have support from your manager [or] Directors, [then] 'I cover my butt'. I do what I have to do. The caseworker judge the manager, the manager judge the caseworker, the caseworker judges the family. And the managers get judged by their managers, and the managers get judged by the Director. The Director's judged by the Minister. In this job, you disempowering clients. I don't think anyone can fix DoCS in my life time. [CW_NESB]

Given the gravity of intervention on families, and because child protection systems would rather *'cover their butt'*, the risk of institutional racism is greater than failing to protect a maltreated child in the name of cultural safety. In other words, the ethical principle of justice – where benefits and risks should be borne and distributed equally across groups – is currently not in play for ethnic minorities. These trends call for a need to relax the level of vigilance in child protection work and thoroughly ensure that removal is justified, but the injustice should also be kept in mind as caseworkers try to resolve the debate between cultural absolutism and cultural relativism.

Resolving them

'Professionals face the debate as to whether child abuse is relative or absolute' (Westby, 2007, p. 144), and struggle with how to implement it in the field. 'Distinguishing cultural differences from child maltreatment is also hampered in large part because child protection workers are usually restricted to problematic individuals and families rather than to the full continuum of acceptable and unacceptable behaviours' (Korbin, 2008, p. 125).

Because of the complexity associated with culture and child protection, caseworkers are at risk of swinging between the two end points of the 'absolutist– relativist' pendulum in their work (Harran, 2002). At one point, they may take a 'universal' stance, and at other times be above all else sensitive to cultural nuance. This swinging renders their fundamental approach towards working with ethnic minority families inconsistent, and therefore outcomes to ethnic minority children and families inconsistent. And if each caseworker is swinging, then the risks of institutional racism and child safety are multiplied. Only lucky families who happen to have a caseworker high on cultural competency will benefit from a good service, rendering the system's capacity to deal with culture inefficient.

Overall then, an emphasis on either absolutism or relativism is dire for the ethnic minority child and 'both, unmoderated, can lead to the misidentification of child maltreatment' (Korbin, 2008, p. 123). One approach to address this is to take an absolutist approach to diagnosis and a relativist approach to delivery. As Westby (2007) puts it:

> Children's best interest[s] (regardless of their cultural background) are best served by adopting an absolutist approach to the diagnosis and recognition of abuse, focusing on the experience of the child rather than the intent of the caregivers, but employing a relativistic approach in determining the types of services to be provided once it is recognised.
>
> (p. 144)

This approach is child-centred, fundamental to good practice given that the role of child protection workers and systems is to protect children from harm, regardless of their cultural background, but it also lives up to its onus to deliver intervention in a culturally appropriate way:

We have to be culturally sensitive, understand [their] background, be flexible when we're getting them engaged with our service [and] involved with case management. [But] when it comes to making a decision, it is by law. Child protection issues override any other cultural issues. Our law is our standard, and we have to justify ourselves against those laws. [CW_NESB]

Our primary focus needs to always be the safety of the child. Although you understand the cultural issues, you can't guarantee the child's safety based on those beliefs and the intention behind [them]. To do that, you're placing the child at risk. Sometimes, you can see where the family's coming from, what they were trying to achieve, [and] just because that doesn't fit into Anglo society, it doesn't mean that it's completely incorrect. But if you've made recommendations that the child stay in their parents' care, based on your familiarity with that culture rather than [on] the child's safety, and [then] something happens to that child, yeah, [you have to] weigh it up. [CW_NESB]

This approach is in line with Koramoa *et al.* (2002), who advocate for some middle ground between absolutist and culturally relative concepts of abuse, and Irfan and Cowburn (2004) who argue that some sort of absolute standard line, which if crossed indicates abuse or neglect, is necessary in child protection practice to avoid the pitfalls of cultural relativism and help ensure that all children are protected from harm. The limitation of this approach, however, is that it does not guarantee overcoming the issue that some behaviours are both culturally acceptable and harmful. It only 'works' when the line that determines whether a behaviour has 'gone beyond what is acceptable crosses not just what is unacceptable in the mainstream culture, but also in the culture of the group in question' (Chand, 2000, cited in Harran, 2002, p. 411).

This limitation reveals a fundamental problem with trying to find a 'balance between ethnocentrism and cultural relativism, core to understanding which aspects of a family's strengths or difficulties are cultural, which are abusive or neglectful and which are a combination of factors' (Korbin, 2008, p. 122). The tension between cultural absolutism and cultural relativism is an *inherent* one, and inherent tensions, by definition, cannot be reconciled. Trying to empirically resolve how to balance child safety with respect for cultural differences in parenting is futile, and accepting that this tension is inherent to child protection work in multicultural countries is a progressive step towards delivering culturally competent service. In other words, a 'middle ground or middle line' does not actually exist; it too is subjective to try and identify:

Where to draw that line? It's so subjective. [CW_Anglo]

Where do you draw the line between being culturally sensitive, and being fair, being just? Because if you go beyond that line, technically you're not being fair toward the Anglo Australian, because [then] are you doing this because they're a different skin colour? If you do that, it's not fair for the other person. [CW_NESB]

Thus, best practice ultimately occurs at the case-by-case level, and culturally appropriate needs can only at best be used heuristically. As a result, a better approach to avoiding the swing between absolutism and relativism than finding some general place in the middle is to be fully educated and aware of the risks that absolutism and relativism each carry: only then caseworkers will be in an informed position to do what is best for a particular ethnic minority child. Just knowing what could go wrong with either approach *is* the approach that needs to be taken. It is the best defence against running, downplaying or minimising their risks, and it is a simple guiding principle that allows for tailoring to unique needs. It better reflects the need for a 'sophisticated relationship between the two moral positions' (Cowan *et al.*, 2001, p. 27). The overall effect is that it protects children from harm, and equally across cultures.

To put it all another way, taking an absolutist position towards the diagnosis of maltreatment does not dodge the issue that diagnostic criteria still depend on cultural norms, and (i) the power of the mainstream to maintain their cultural norms is usually greater than the power of minority groups, in which case it would further perpetuate the injustice of risks and benefits being unequally borne by ethnic minorities, or (ii) that even if groups are treated as equals, they differ in what they see as harmful and acceptable, in which case, who is right? Really, the answer to this question is the child's state. If the outcome of a behaviour is detrimental to a child's well-being, then harm can be said to have occurred and intervention is justified. Herein lies the importance of child-centred practice. However, although child-centred practice is a principle that should fundamentally guide child protection work, it too needs to be implemented in culturally sensitive and respectful ways to be effective with ethnic minority families. In short, both diagnosis and delivery require relativism, not just delivery.

Implementing child-centred practice effectively with ethnic minority families

So far, it has been established that culturally appropriate diagnostic criteria are required for accurate assessments to avoid the great risk of ethnocentricism on ethnic minorities. Doing so, also takes a child-centred approach because it does not inappropriately separate the child's cultural and cultural safety needs from their other safety needs.

A child-centred approach to child welfare lies at the heart of the United Nations (UN) Hague Convention on the Rights of the Child (CRC). The UN CRC (1989) includes: the right to survival; the right to development of their full physical and mental potential; the right to protection from influences that are harmful to their development; and the right to participation in family, cultural and social life (cited in Westby, 2007, p. 142).

According to Cahn (2002), 'the willingness to focus on the individual child reflects much broader social, legal and philosophical notions about the child as a future deserving citizen of the state, who is valuable regardless of the suitability or desirability of his or her parents' (p. 481). In the context of child protection, 'it is of paramount importance for social care services to remain child-centred if they are to prevent children being abused or exposed to danger' (Harran, 2002, p. 413).

To ensure that the child's safety remains at the forefront of decision-making about their best interests (Thomson and Molloy, 2001), regardless of their cultural background, Maitra (2005) notes that 'attribution of responsibility does not require evidence of intention to cause harm, and that parental care is judged on the basis of whether it has been adequate or has caused harm' (p. 255). Similarly, Chan *et al.* (2002) argues that the child protection system should focus on the experience of and outcomes for children, rather than the intent of the caregiver, as this approach offers better protection against cross-cultural misunderstanding (cited in Westby, 2007).

Although child-centred practice remains the key principle for child protection policies and practices (Winkworth and McArthur, 2006), it is a practice that '*de-centres* the parent' (McConnell and Llewellyn, 2005). While challenging to all families, it is particularly challenging to collectivist families.

It is challenging to all families because it represents a dilemma between the rights of parents to determine how to raise their children and the rights of children to be safe (Westby, 2007). Indeed, 'child abuse and neglect statutes are premised on the concept that parents' basic rights become attenuated as soon as the fitness of the parents becomes questionable' (Cahn, 2002, p. 479). This is consistent with a notion that parents should more be seen as having the *responsibility* to care for their child's safety, as compared to a *right* to care for their children. Such a shift would be consistent with Harran's (2002) assertion 'that the necessary cultural shift is in valuing all children' (cited in Gough and Lynch, 2002, p. 343). For example, Cahn (2002) notes that 'the tension between what is best for the child and the cultural parameters of good families appears in the child welfare system where remaining in a biological family may mean that a child stays with an undeserving mother' (p. 470).

Arguably, the tension can be attenuated by upholding child-centred practice and keeping the child's safety at the centre of all decision-making, by redefining the dilemma: the debate should not be centred around whether parents have the right to care for their own children, but whether children have the right to be cared for by their own parents. In other words, decision-making processes about the best interests of a child should re-conceptualise the tension as not between child and parent, but between two of the child's own conflicting needs and rights – the right to be protected from harm and the right to be cared for by their own parents. Thus, parents would have a *responsibility* to care for their children well, and children would have a *right* to be cared for by their parents well. This view would also meet the call by Sidebotham (2013) that child protection systems be 'authoritative' in the same way they expect parents to be authoritative – combining the provision of care and (earned) control.

This would change the child-centred approach to a 'child-centred and family-focused' approach to child protection because both rights of children would be acknowledged. Thus, if significant harm was substantiated – their right to be safe from harm was violated – then their other right to be cared for by their parents would also need to be seriously weighed against the trauma that would be incurred to children by removing them from their family; it would not *just* be about substantiation of serious maltreatment.

Of course, caseworkers already do this in practice – they care about what is best for the child by considering if it is better to keep children within their home, while taking into account the frequency and severity of maltreatment. For example, caseworkers involved in the NSW Children's Court need to make assessments based on the 'balance of probabilities'; those that assess the relative strengths or weaknesses of a decision to keep a child within or remove a child from their family, and in keeping with the best practice principle to keep families together. However, the call for a 'child-centred and family-focused' approach to child protection here is more about formalising the decision-making process, so that both rights of children are equally represented. Indeed, one caseworker said:

> There is a difference between the 'child's best interests' and the 'best interests of the child'. One is determined by adults, and one determined by children. *[CW_ANON]*

Examples of good practice 2.5 –
Child-centred practice with inclusion of children's voices

Clinical psychologist report: Her preference to stay in her family needs to be acknowledged and respected by external authorities as to do otherwise could well be experienced by the child as a repetition of her mother's dismissal of her wishes and opinions. [VIE_case file]

It should be noted that although the child has frequently indicated a vehement desire to return to his parents' care during conversation with me, he has also expressed a firm wish that they would 'stop hitting' him. 'They hit me for everything.' [CHN_case file]

Similarly, Parton (2009) argues that the current system is in fact 'adult-centric' despite claiming that it is child-centric. Thus, if child-centred practice really values children, then all the needs and rights of children must really be valued; 'the very real pain caused by separating children from their families should not be minimised. The damage caused by disrupting these ties may be far greater than the harm agencies are trying to avoid' (Roberts, 2003, p. 173):

This is the conflict I have. We remove the children, not work with the parents. DoCS are extremely unique in this approach. DoCS [are] more child-focused as opposed to family-focused. [CW_NESB]

For us, it's about maintaining the bottom line of child safety. Whilst we talk the rhetoric of trying to keep families together, ultimately what it means is as long as the kids are safe. We are often disempowering people even further around [their] choices, 'you need to enforce an AVO, you need to do this, you need to do that, because if you don't, you are potentially going to lose your children'. We are forcing [their] hand. That's a dilemma in any family. [CW_Anglo]

I often find that a quandary myself – about how can you be child-focused without looking at the family that children belong [to]? There is a real need to place emphasis on looking at it from the child's eyes because they are often the voiceless ones in this equation, and it is easy to get absorbed in the parents, but really, who can draw a line between 'child-focus'? You can't separate it from working in a family context. I call it 'containing the containers'. In looking after the parents you are actually looking after the children. [CW_Anglo]

A 'child-centred and family-focused approach' also addresses the issue that ethnic minority families tend to originate from collectivist cultures, and in such cultures, overt hierarchical structures are normative, acceptable and of value. For example, males have more social power than females and older people have more social power than younger people. A 'child-centred approach' to child welfare is essential for the protection of children, but is more aligned and sits more comfortably with individualism, because it requires turning upside-down the social structures of collectivist families, giving more power to children than is usual:

Looking at cultural and moral beliefs from other countries/religions, [there is] a difference in cultural values placed on the worth of the child's right to be a child. That is not in line with NSW legislation or the Hague Convention. Western countries tend to have different societal views on the life of children, and their right to protection. [CW_Anglo]

NM said the incident with son was 'very minor'. NM would never seriously harm the child – she loves the kids. Child has become 'a little monster' and 'mr untouchable'. Blames the Department for giving child so much power. He wasn't like that before Dept got involved. From the first contact with CW, he became a different person. Feels they became 'hostages' after child's meeting with CW as he would threaten to call DoCS if anything happens. [CHN_case file]

Even though they are there for my children, they have to understand that they spend a few hours with [them]. When they leave, I am the one who's going to spend 24 hours with the children [and] clean up after their mess that's going to be affected by the way they behave. So they have also to look after me, consider me, where I come from, who I am. I know DoCS apply the law, and I don't think they're going to consider my point of view, but if they were to, I would suggest they should also listen to the parents, give a chance to the parents to explain themselves and give their side of the story, pay [them] more attention. [FAM_Burundian]

I can say for all Sudanese, we [are] having big problems with DoCS. When we bring up our children, it need just parents. We're trying to integrate, trying to learn English, but our children, they don't have English background, so they like to speak out, but they know nothing. They don't have [the] meanings of words. So sometimes our children say wrong thing and this will reflect their family. It's the biggest problem in our community. If your child ring police, then police ring DoCS, they come straight away, and do their job, without your information, without any permission from you. That's the major problem with the parents. Culturally, it's not ok, especially children under 12. And if we try to control our kids, you know, not talk to people, it will look like we're preventing them for integration, so we getting confused now... [If] DoCS receive that child for [a] few months or few years, they let her go and then [they] become a street boy or street girl. These are the crimes that are now raising at the moment. Our community is aware of that, and we're trying to say something on it. [FAM_Sudanese]

The literature makes similar points. 'Children in the Middle East, and particularly sons, have always been valued and socialised into specific gender roles, including the division of labour, at an early age. There is little evidence of a carefree childhood or of childhood as an important stage in itself' (Makhoul *et al.*, 2003, p. 249). Shalhoub-Kevorkian (2005) also says, 'Western society's construction of child abuse differs from the politics of child abuse in non-Western societies. In China, familism (success, unity and reputation of the family), and filial piety (the expectation that children are subordinate to the wishes of their parents) are adhered to at the expense of the individual' (p. 1265). As a result, 'the traditional Confucian ethic of filial piety is sometimes interpreted as a dictate that children must be unquestioningly loyal and obedient to their parents and look after their parents' needs' (Kim *et al.*, 2006, p. 371).

In short, collectivist ethnic minorities experience particular challenges in Western child protection systems. Their cultural conceptualisations of the family and child-rearing, in which parents overtly have more power than their children and children are less seen as individual units than they are as members of the family group, which is more important, are challenged by child-centred practice to child welfare in Western countries that abide by the UN CRC.

A 'child-centred and family-focused' approach to child welfare would benefit all families, regardless of their cultural background. However, it would also help intervention be more culturally appropriate with ethnic minorities, for whom overt power structures within the family yield children at the bottom of the hierarchy. The current 'child-centred approach' is more consistent with individualistic values, in which there is an overt striving for more vertical or equal power relationships among family members, creating problems for effective implementation of a child-centred framework for collectivist families.

Moreover, 'culture can bring with it both risk and protective factors, whose impact varies not only between cultures but also within any culture, and cultural competency intervention and treatment should focus not only on pathological behaviours that can be labelled maltreatment but equally importantly on cultural strength that can mitigate risk' (Korbin, 2008, p. 128); 'deficits in cultural competency may have devastating effects on safeguarding children from harm' (Harran, 2002, p. 411). The most important strength that collectivists have as a protective factor in times of family dysfunction is cohesion. For example, Suaalii and Mavoa (2001) note that:

> The tension between the individual and collective is highlighted in policies for children and young people which have been developed from the eurocentric values and beliefs embedded in the constitutional and political systems of New Zealand. In Pacific communities, the rights of children in extended families are collectively framed, knowledge is collectively owned and 'life stage' is privileged over age.
>
> (p. 39)

Family cohesion and togetherness, despite infrequent and/or chronic (as opposed to acute) maltreatment, are crucial for the development of a child's well-being, regardless of their cultural background. As Harris and Hackett (2008) point out, 'when a child has to be separated from their parent/s either temporarily or permanently, this experience is emotionally traumatic for the child as well as the birth parents' (p. 211):

> *I was totally upset when they removed my son. I start being happy when I received my son. If you compare the problems that you face back home and the problem you dealing with now, no different. [FAM_Sudanese]*

However, among strongly collectivistic ethnic minority groups – in which family cohesion is the focal point around which family life revolves – the extent of this trauma may be intensified considerably. That is, the extent to which family cohesion acts as a protective factor, and should be regarded as a strength among these families, protecting or mitigating against infrequent and/or chronic maltreatment, should not be under-estimated. In fact, Cahn (2002) points out of all families, 'even after substantiation of abuse or neglect, studies have found that the majority of children in OOHC could safely live at home' (p. 477). However, such trends may be contextualised for ethnic minorities as the result of the protection that strong family cohesion offers.

This idea for a 'child-centred and family-focused' approach to child welfare is not new (e.g. Kriẑ and Skivenes, 2012; Parkinson, 2003; Sandau-Beckler *et al.*, 2002). Roberts (1997) long ago acknowledged that black children in the USA should be protected from neglect and abuse, and sometimes even removed from their homes, but nevertheless argues that it is in fact a violation of children's rights to remove them from their families of origin; 'the solution is not to remove children from their parents, but to provide support so that their parents can raise their own children, and not through their involvement with a (institutionally) racially biased system' (cited in Cahn, 2002, p. 481). As Shalhoub-Kevorkian (2005) puts it, 'state intervention in the family life of an already-oppressed group leaves children vulnerable to all forms of abuse, including abuses that are direct consequences of formal interventions' (p. 1266). Even more recently, Featherstone *et al.* (2014) say that 'the current child-centric risk paradigm is highly problematic ethically. It is wedded to constructions of children as individuals who are unanchored in networks and communities' (p. 16).

Contrarily, Bartholet (1999) advocates that children should be removed and placed for adoption (or other temporary and longer-term placements) more quickly because of potential or actual harm, and that protection of their parents should not be at the core of an abuse and neglect system (cited in Cahn, 2002). Bartholet (1999) critiques the 'blood bias' of the current system, which strives to keep children with their parents or within their kinship group, and argues that parenting should be defined by 'social', not blood-based bonds. She argues that 'it is important to move African American children into other homes where they will receive the nurturing they need, rather than leaving them with their biological parents' (cited in Cahn, 2002, p. 478). She holds these views on the grounds that racial disproportionality (or over-representation) in the child protection system is warranted; African American children experience more maltreatment due to higher exposure to risk factors like poverty (Bartholet, 2009).

A view in favour of removal makes several errors of judgement. First, it assumes that failing to remove children at risk of harm is somehow siding with parents; that a 'blood-bond' bias is parent-focused, not child-centred. So long as the risk of harm is not significant, it is actually siding with the child to keep them with their family; family cohesion is in the child's best interest. Second, it exemplifies how the protective strength of family cohesion is or can be under-estimated for strongly kinship or community-based groups. For example, in individualistic cultures, 'too much' family cohesion may be seen as a problem in the family rather than a strength because self-sufficiency is highly regarded and valued as a protective factor (Forehand and Kotchick, 2002), and also because families from individualistic cultures may perceive that families from collectivistic cultures place the needs of adults and elders above the needs of the child. Third, it assumes that, as a rule, non-biological caregivers, such as foster carers, are 'nurturing'. Of course, several are, but this view heuristically assumes that the nurturing that good foster carers provide exceeds the warmth offered from blood bonds (see also Chapter 9). Indeed, the 'rule of optimism' – or the focus on an adult's strengths leading to under-responsiveness (Dingwall *et al.*, 2014) – is also criticised, and by corollary, so should it here too. Finally, it seems driven by the need to provide an 'ideal' home for a child, rather than prevent maltreatment, and Maitra (2005) warns against assuming needs as universal and needs being synonymous with ideals. (Having said that, the conditions that constitute a 'good enough' parent – with minimal parenting competence – also need to be explicitly identified; Choate and Engstrom, 2014.) As has been noted for Indigenous families, 'whole kinship families are affected by the wounds of invasion and (only) "whole of family" therapy can assist recovery and strengthen the "circles of care" around the child'.[4]

Certainly, the welfare of children, and not the parents, is at the heart of any risk assessment. However, unless the abuse or neglect is so severe that it is, without a doubt, necessary to remove the child from their abusive or neglectful family environment, and that 'blood ties' do not in any way justify keeping the child with these abusive or neglectful caregivers, the general rule of thumb for all families (not just ethnic minorities) should be to keep the family together, and intervention should be focused on parental education and support rather than termination of parental *responsibilities*.

Even in families with complex needs, where it is likely that 'concerns fall into more than one of the categories – physical, sexual or emotional abuse and neglect' (Chand and Thoburn, 2006, p. 369), support should target the specific issues causing stress to the family, such as domestic violence, mental health issues or substance abuse rehabilitation. Indeed, 'lack of access to (formal or informal) childcare or insufficient knowledge about community services or alternative forms of disciplining children and parenting guidance compound these problems' (Giglio, 1997, p. 6) and should be the focus of intervention.

Of the system in the USA, Cahn (2002) points out that:

> Over the past 30 years the child protective services system has focused on removal at the expense of preservation; the number of children receiving in-home services declined by 60% from 1977 to 1994. Such a restructuring might make clients more comfortable seeking and accepting preservation services if they know they are getting help rather than confronting a high risk of child removal. A broader vision of child welfare services would involve support for children's existing needy families and less focus on punishing those families.
>
> (p. 477)

Collectivist families 'strongly resist interference in family lives by outsiders because family affairs, especially with regard to child-rearing practices, are considered strictly the family's own business. The family is regarded as a private realm, beyond the control of both the state and the politics' (Hahm and Guterman, 2001, p. 174). This makes it especially important for ethnic minorities to feel 'safe' that statutory child protection workers are there to assist their family, rather than to remove their children. In turn, they will be more likely to report maltreatment and seek useful assistance (Maiter *et al.*, 2004).

Support in the form of education is also required. Focusing on the child's outcomes of a parenting behaviour and not of the intent behind it, to promote insight into its harmful effects, should be the basis for engaging in a 'child-centred and family-focused' way with families:

> *Explain to the family the common ground – that we [both] want what's best for the children. [CW_NESB]*

> *The first thing is that all children have the right to feel safe. If you come from that perspective, and you put it to families, everyone understands that. That's the best way to start a conversation with any family, 'we have something in common. I'm working because I want your child to be safe'. No one will disagree. [CW_NESB]*

Emphasising that child safety is the common ground between parents and authorities is a good way forward in terms of implementing child-centred practice with (collectivist and all) families that otherwise de-centres the parent.

Key points

- The main risk associated with cultural absolutism (the use of ethnocentric assessment tools) is greater for ethnic minorities than the risks with cultural relativism (permitting harm in the name of respect of cultural diversity and failing to diagnose maltreatment) because the institutional culture of 'it's better to be safe than sorry' tilts the swing; the focal point of the debate is not just about child safety, it is also about protecting the institution's liability.
- To avoid swinging between the 'absolutist–relativist' pendulum, caseworkers should be fully aware of and educated on the pitfalls of both stances towards child protection work in culturally diverse communities, and apply them on a subjective and case-by-case basis. The two points represent the ends of an inherent tension, and so education is the only and best defence against them both; trying to heuristically resolve them is futile. The diagnosis of maltreatment and delivery of culturally appropriate intervention are complex, so it is best to start with the child, and use a child-centred approach.
- Child-centred practice (consistent with the UN CRC) is essential for determining the safety of a child and their best interests, but is challenging to implement with families because it requires de-centring the parent, and particularly challenging with collectivist families in which children overtly and normatively have lower social power than elders.

Recommendations for practice

✓   Review and revise risk of harm assessment tools to ensure items are culturally appropriate. Validate these tools by consulting with local ethnic community groups.

✓   The extent to which children have a right to be cared for by their parents should be given formal consideration; and parents should be seen as having a responsibility to care for their children, not a right.

✓   The extent to which family cohesion acts as a protective factor, mitigating risks to a child's safety, should not be under-estimated or overlooked in assessments of collectivist families. Imposing individualistic norms and values about self-sufficiency, over family dependency, pathologises collectivist cultures for valuing the family over the child. It also aids the use of a 'child-centred and family-focused' approach to child welfare.

✓   Unless harm is significant and removal is justified, supporting and educating parents to develop insight, rather than punishing and disempowering vulnerable families, is the best means of protecting children from harm.

Notes

1   www.aija.org.au/TherapJurisp06/Papers/Nethercott%20%20PPT.pdf
2   About one-quarter of all children in the NSW child protection system are Indigenous.
3   Of Australia's population, 33 per cent are born overseas and 24 per cent are born in non-English speaking countries (ABS 3412.0, 2007a). In order, the largest ethnic minority groups in Australia are from Italy, China, Vietnam, India, the Philippines, Greece, Germany, South Africa, Malaysia, the Netherlands, Lebanon and Hong Kong (ABS 1301.0, 2007b).
4   www.aija.org.au/TherapJurisp06/Papers/Nethercott%20%20PPT.pdf

Part II
Practice issues

3 Frequency of maltreatment

What are the most common types of abuse and neglect reported across cultures and what is their effect on children?

Primary and secondary types of abuse and neglect reported across cultures

A recent study in the UK suggests that the prevalence of child maltreatment is reducing (Radford *et al.*, 2011). However, ascertaining the true prevalence of maltreatment is difficult (Ferrari, 2002). As Clark (1995) says:

> Child protection data from the UK, USA and (Australian) states tell a similar story – the statistics reveal more about the ambiguous definition of child abuse and neglect, and the anxiety of the community and professional groups, than they do about real incidence; child protection data measure the investigative and administrative work-loads of the agencies involved.
>
> (p. 23)

It becomes even more difficult in communities where there is strong pressure to keep family matters private, making it seem that the prevalence of child maltreatment is lower in ethnic minority communities. As an example:

> To many Chinese, the family is still a private sphere. Public authorities do not usually intervene because the heavy emphasis on filial piety forbids children to complain against their parents; family shames should be kept within the confines of the family, and the public are not inclined to intrude into the private domain of the family to avoid shattering it. As a result, many cases of child maltreatment may escape public attention, giving the impression that child maltreatment is a very rare phenomenon in China.
>
> (Qiao and Chan, 2005, p. 24)

Mandatory reporting is changing this somewhat:

> *I've been working here for about eight or nine years. In [that] time, I've noticed a massive shift in the reports we are receiving around CALD groups. Back then, we weren't receiving many reports, so they weren't as predominant within our child protection system. [But] with mandatory reporting, more*

communities [are] coming through. It is becoming more apparent. It is not as hidden as before. [CW_NESB]

**Example of poor practice 3.1 –
Over-estimating the prevalence of maltreatment in ethnic minority communities**

We have five or six Muslim-identified schools in this area. We rarely get reports from [them so] we don't really know what's going on. We know that abuse is fairly rife in those cultures but we don't get reports, which I think is a huge cultural issue. They're saying they're mandatory reporters, however it's [abuse] acceptable in their culture [so] they turn a blind eye. If you did a project in there, I reckon half those children would end up getting removed. [CW_Anglo]

Overall, however, cultural pressures to keep family matters private make it difficult to ascertain the true prevalence of child maltreatment in ethnic minority communities; reporting biases are significant and need to be adequately taken into account (and no more). However, the prevalence of each *type* of maltreatment across cultures can be more accurately gauged after reporting and entry into the child protection system.

To do this, each case file was reviewed for all the types of abuse and neglect reported in it. Importantly, an equal (but small) number of case files per cultural group, which were all randomly selected, means that the quantitative data in this study approaches representativeness; the prevalence of each type of maltreatment in this sample likely reflects the population. A replication study with larger samples per cultural group would be required to conduct statistical analyses and confirm the findings.

The three main types of *abuse* scoped for were (i) physical, (ii) sexual and (iii) emotional, and the three main types of *neglect* were (i) neglect of basic needs, (ii) educational neglect and (iii) inadequate supervision. These six categories were identified as appropriate by caseworkers who took part in a validation study to ensure that the Thematic Template that case files would be reviewed against was comprehensive and relevant.

Of all the different types of abuse or neglect reported in a case file, one was deemed the primary type of maltreatment. This was defined as the *most frequently* reported type. If there were two or more equally occurring types of maltreatment, then the most recent or *current* type was deemed the primary type. Sexual abuse or assault was, as a rule, deemed the primary type when other types of abuse or neglect were also reported (e.g. physical or emotional abuse), except in the case where only sexual risk of harm (ROH) was reported (e.g. exposure to pornographic material) but not sexual assault or abuse. All other types of reported maltreatment were deemed secondary types.

In a small number of case files (n=3/120), not enough or no information was provided in the notes to make a decision about the primary or secondary type/s of maltreatment. This points to another kind of reporting bias that can occur – lack of consistency across caseworkers in the identification of all types of abuse and neglect for a child. The risk of this reporting bias is seen as moderate, because risk of harm assessments are definitively driven by the need to identify all types of maltreatment but this does not also guarantee that that occurs; some types of maltreatment may end up being underreported.

Notwithstanding the smaller sample size and reporting biases that can occur among caseworkers, the data in Figure 3.1 shows that physical abuse is the most common primary type among ethnic minorities, and sexual abuse is the most common primary type among Aboriginals and Anglos. These key findings are discussed in Chapter 4. (Note: Educational neglect was not deemed the primary type of maltreatment in any of the case files.)

Figure 3.2 contains information on the secondary types of maltreatment reported across all six cultural groups. As there could be several secondary types, a frequency axis has been used instead of a percentage one.

The results mainly show that the most commonly occurring secondary type of maltreatment reported is emotional abuse (n=68/120). For example, emotional abuse not deemed the primary type was reported in 70 per cent of Chinese

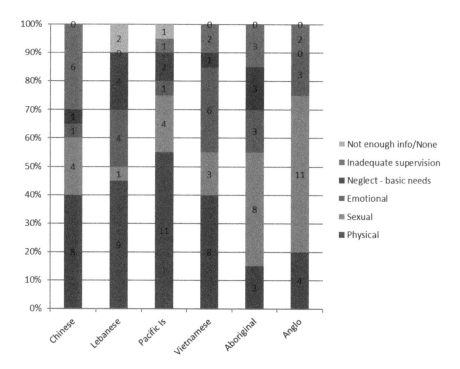

Figure 3.1 Primary type of maltreatment by cultural group

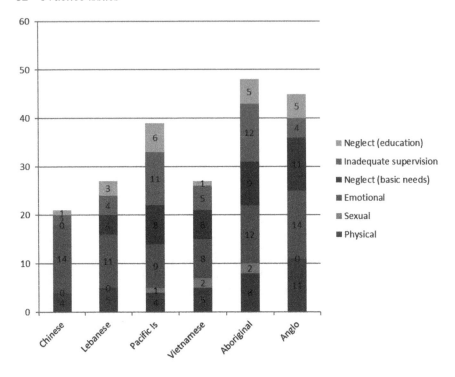

Figure 3.2 Secondary types of maltreatment by cultural group

(n=14/20), 61 per cent of Lebanese (n=11/18), 45 per cent of Pacific Islander (n=9/20), 40 per cent of Vietnamese (n=8/20), 60 per cent of Aboriginal (n=12/20) and 70 per cent of Anglo case files (n=14/20):

> *It's very rare that the primary issue will be emotional abuse and that [that] will be the only factor to lead to a removal. That wouldn't happen. It would just be one factor in that family. [CW_NESB]*

The results also show that physical abuse (n=37/120 cases), neglect of basic needs (n=38/120) and inadequate supervision (n=38/120) were the next most commonly occurring secondary types of maltreatment, and that educational neglect was the least common secondary type of maltreatment reported (n=21/120). Note: sexual risk of harm (but not sexual assault or abuse) was reported in 5/120 case files as a secondary type.

Co-morbidity: number of secondary types of maltreatment

'Co-morbidity' is a borrowed term from medical and psychological literature used here to indicate how many *different* types of maltreatment were reported in each case file. If a child was reported as experiencing only one type (which would have also been the primary type), they would have 'low' (or no) co-morbidity. 'Moderate' (or some) co-morbidity was defined as when a child had two to three different types of maltreatment reported in their case file and 'high' co-morbidity occurred when a child had four to six different types of maltreatment reported in their case file.

Thus, the data on co-morbidity is related to secondary types of maltreatment reported; the more secondary types reported, the greater the co-morbidity. The data on secondary types of maltreatment in Figure 3.2 already shows that co-morbidity is greatest for children of Aboriginal and Anglo background and least for children of Chinese background, but the co-morbidity data in Figure 3.3 (and Data Table 3.1) teases this out more clearly.

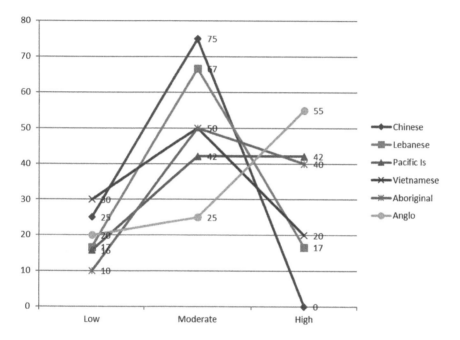

Figure 3.3 Co-morbidity of maltreatment by cultural group

Table 3.1 Co-morbidity of maltreatment by cultural group

	Low (%ᵃ)	*Moderate (%)*	*High (%)*	*Total (%)*
Chinese	5 (25)	15 (75)	0 (0)	20 (100)
Lebanese	3 (17)	12 (67)	3 (17)	18[1] (100)
Pacific Is	3 (16)	8 (42)	8 (42)	19[2] (100)
Vietnamese	6 (30)	10 (50)	4 (20)	20 (100)
Aboriginal	2 (10)	10 (50)	8 (40)	20 (100)
Anglo	4 (20)	5 (25)	11 (55)	20 (100)
Total	23	60	34	117

ᵃ – Row (not column) percentage.

Figure 3.3 shows that for children of Chinese, Lebanese and Vietnamese backgrounds, co-morbidity resembles a bell-curve or normal distribution, with the majority reporting a moderate number of different abuses or neglect (n=2–3), and the remainder reporting either an isolated type of maltreatment (n=1) or a high number of different types of maltreatment (n=4–6). Of note, within these three groups, children of Vietnamese backgrounds report the least variation, as their curve is 'flatter' than the other two groups.

On the other hand, children of Pacific Islander and Aboriginal backgrounds had similar curves, which did not resemble a bell-curve. Their curves indicate that co-morbidity is skewed towards the higher end, with a relatively equal number of reports of 'moderate' and 'high' co-morbidity for each group. That is, the number of children with two to three types of maltreatment and the number of children with four to six types of maltreatment were both high and relatively equal.

Finally, children of Anglo background had the most unique curve, with no resemblance to their counterparts. Co-morbidity for this group appeared neither statistically normal in the way it was for families of Chinese, Lebanese and Vietnamese backgrounds, nor did it grow at the moderate and higher ends in the way it did for families of Pacific Islander and Aboriginal backgrounds. The majority of Anglo children are reported to experience four to six different types of maltreatment; fewer Anglo children are reported to experience one to three different types of maltreatment. Thus, for example, physical abuse may be reported as the only issue for an ethnic minority child, but for an Anglo child, this type of abuse is more likely to be one of several other types that the child is also reported to be experiencing.

These results indicate one of two possibilities. On the one hand, it could be an accurate reflection of dysfunction, suggesting that children of Anglo, Aboriginal and Pacific Islander backgrounds tend to experience four to six different types of maltreatment, and that children of Chinese, Lebanese and Vietnamese backgrounds tend to experience one to three different types of maltreatment. This possibility is corroborated by one caseworker who said:

> *I think Anglo groups are harder to work with. They've got more issues, like drug and alcohol, mental health, domestic violence compared to the migrants and CALD groups I work with. [CW_NESB]*

Alternatively, the results occur because the bias of lack of consistency across caseworkers in identifying all the types of maltreatment a child may be experiencing is systematically related to the child's ethnicity. Theoretically, if there is under-reporting of maltreatment due to this reporting bias, then it would be equally spread across groups, boosting merit for the first possibility – that dysfunction really is greater and more diverse in some cultural groups than others (and if anything, that Anglo children should be as over-represented in the child protection system as Aboriginal children).

However, it is possible that since there are fewer ethnic minority children in the child protection system compared to Aboriginal and Anglo children, there may be less exposure to individual variation among ethnic minorities and thus greater reliance on stereotypes while making assessments. For example, disproportionate attention may be given to physical abuse if it is substantiated because it is stereotypically consistent for ethnic minorities, minimising attention to other types of maltreatment that may also be occurring within a family. Indeed, Shalhoub-Kevorkian (2005) points out that 'data from the United States reveal similar sexual, physical and emotional child abuse across different ethnic groups, yet there are still prejudices and stereotypes regarding minority and certain ethnic groups' (p. 1266). More research on this is required. As a practice issue, however, these findings point to the necessity of standardising assessment of *all* types of maltreatment for *all* children.

The effect of abuse and neglect on children

Regardless of the type of maltreatment, children who are abused or neglected suffer greatly. The case files showed that regardless of a child's cultural background, behavioural and mental health issues were the most common effects of maltreatment (described in more detail below), and to a lesser extent that conflict with parents (e.g. normal conflict common during adolescence, conflict due to cultural differences across generations, etc.), absconding (e.g. running away from home, truanting from school, etc.), sexualised behaviour (e.g. inappropriate sexual behaviour towards brother, older and seductive appearance, etc.), being identified as a high-needs child, criminal activity and physical health issues (e.g. underweight, obesity, hyper-insulinism, scabies, asthma, eczema, golden staph, etc.) are also reported (see Table 3.2).

Behavioural issues sometimes overlapped with criminal activity and included:

- *violence or aggression* (e.g. assaulting mother, abusing people in the street, violent tendencies displayed to younger siblings, lighting fires, impulsivity, risk-taking behaviours, defiance and non-compliance, property damage and shoplifting/stealing, etc.);
- *erratic, withdrawn and/or challenging behaviour* (e.g. losing temper easily, defensive and argumentative if they do not get their way, children reacting to blaming, accusations and bullying, no respect towards police or authority, etc.);
- *problems at school* (e.g. chronic disobedience, inappropriate language, uncooperative with staff, aggressive with other children, not accepted by students in peer group, often in trouble, throwing tantrums and running away from school, suspended for hitting other school children, threatening to kill others including principal, etc.);
- *problems at childcare* (e.g. banned from childcare, difficult behaviour, always in trouble for pushing, hitting and shoving other children, etc.).

Summarily, the wide range of mental health issues reported across all case files included: attention deficit hyperactivity disorder (ADHD), oppositional defiant

Table 3.2 Presentations of maltreated children by cultural group

	Chinese	Lebanese	Pacific Is	Vietnamese	Aboriginal	Anglo	Total
Behavioural issues	6	6	4	2	6	5	29
Mental health issues	6	2	4	5	5	5	27
Conflict with parents[3]	6	2	7	4	2	1	22
Absconding (runaways)	0	1	4	2	4	7	18
Sexualised behaviour	0	1	1	1	4	4	11
High-needs child	1	0	3	1	4	2	11
Criminal activity	0	0	3	0	3	0	6
Physical health issues	0	0	2	0	2	0	4
Total	19	12	28	15	30	24	

disorder (ODD), obsessive compulsive disorder (OCD), conduct disorder, reactive attachment disorder (RAD), post-traumatic stress disorder (PTSD), schizophrenia, anxiety disorders, high emotionality and irrationality, depression (including prescriptions for antidepressants), self-harming behaviour, threat to self-harm (e.g. head banging, threats to kill themselves) and suicidal ideation. One *"mother called to say her child is pregnant and returned home once with stab wounds to her stomach and back which were self-inflicted" [ABR_case file]*. Thus, mental health issues vary in intensity and can be severe.

Overall, if evidence of poor outcomes like behavioural and mental health issues is found, this should be part of the conversation with parents when trying to develop their insight into the harmful effects of their parenting behaviour, regardless of their intention. This is consistent with the approach that education to promote insight, and focusing on the child's outcomes of behaviour, should be the basis for culturally appropriate engagement with ethnic minority (and all) families (see Chapter 2 on 'child-centred, family focused' intervention).

It is even more critical with ethnic minorities, who may resist seeking support and services for their mentally ill children due to the stigma associated with mental illness and the cultural pressure to protect the family name:

> *Cultural factors may have contributed to NM's unwillingness to accept that her daughter had a mental health problem and to ask for assistance. [CHN_case file]*

> *Child was diagnosed with early onset schizophrenia and a report from hospital suggests that the delay in child receiving treatment [NM refused*

treatment for 10 months] worsened the impact of her condition. [CHN_case file]

In some cases, not seeking appropriate supports is considered medical neglect (see Chapter 4). Of course, some families do access services, highlighting why it is important not to stereotype families:

NF has responded appropriately to child's mental health concerns. Has made significant changes to his own life in order to accommodate child's needs and has established relationships with professionals involved in child's care. [CHN_case file]

Key points

- The pressure to keep family matters private may make it seem that maltreatment is less frequent in ethnic minority groups because reports are fewer, even with mandatory reporting. However, prevalence of maltreatment should also not be over-estimated in ethnic minority groups, as this would be racism.
- Overall, the *effects* of abuse and neglect are similar for children across cultures.
  - o Maltreated children may present with behavioural issues, mental health issues, conflict with parents, running away, sexualised behaviour, being identified as a high-needs child, criminal activity and/or physical health issues.
  - o Conflict with parents for ethnic minority children may be partly due to normal developmental conflict during adolescence and partly due to acculturative stress between migrant parents and children.
- Although the effects of maltreatment are not strongly related to culture, the *type* of maltreatment seems to be.
  - o Physical abuse is the most common primary type of maltreatment reported for ethnic minority children.
  - o Sexual abuse is the most common primary type of maltreatment reported for Aboriginal and Anglo children.
- Children of Anglo, Aboriginal and Pacific Islander backgrounds tend to have more *different* types of maltreatment reported (n=4–6).
- Children of Chinese, Lebanese and Vietnamese backgrounds tend to have fewer *different* types of maltreatment reported (n=1–3).
- Either systematic reporting on all the different types of maltreatment for a child may not be equal across cultural groups, or some groups may genuinely have higher co-morbidity of abuse and neglect than others.

Recommendations for practice

To ensure equity in the way assessments of maltreatment are made:

✓ Be mindful not to pay more attention to stereotypically consistent types of maltreatment for ethnic minorities (e.g. physical abuse) over other types.

✓ Improve data accuracy and completeness by standardising assessment fields that caseworkers make decisions on – they should report on both what is and is not present. This way, all data fields will have been considered for all families.

✓ Suggested data fields include:
- o   Types of maltreatment – physical abuse, sexual abuse, emotional abuse, inadequate supervision and neglect of basic needs.
- o   Risk factors of maltreatment – domestic violence, alcohol and other drug issues, mental health issues in carers, poverty and homelessness.
- o   Presentations among maltreated children – behavioural issues, mental health issues, conflict with parents, running away, sexualised behaviour, being identified as a high-needs child, criminal activity and physical health issues.

✓ In light of caseworkers being time-poor, these data fields should be a simple 'tick in the box' indicating the presence of the issue, with opportunity to provide details only on data fields relevant to the child and family.

Notes

1 Two case files did not have sufficient information to make an assessment on primary and secondary types of maltreatment.

2 One case file had no reported issues after an assessment was made. Thus, it is differentiated from case files in which there was insufficient information to determine the primary type of maltreatment.

3 Reports of 'conflict with parents' for ethnic minorities did not always differentiate between its developmental and acculturative components; this depth of analysis would improve assessment and engagement.

4   Culture and maltreatment

Are physical abuse, sexual abuse, emotional abuse, inadequate supervision and neglect of basic needs related to culture?

Physical abuse

Reports of physical abuse were found in the case files from all six cultural groups:

> *Cigarette burns. [PAC_case file]*

> *Hit by step-mother who has thrown chairs and knives at her. [ANG_case file]*

> *Paternal uncle punched child in the stomach and smacked him on the face many times. [LEB_case file]*

> *Mother has physically assaulted child by repeatedly kicking, hitting and punching him with steel capped boots. Child [also] repeatedly choked by his mother. [PAC_case file]*

> *Parents have long history of abuse. Ongoing cruel, physical punishment including standing child outside in the rain at night, leaving him unsupervised in the garage till their return late from work at night. [CHN_case file]*

> *NM admitted to punishing the child by heating a knife over a hot plate and placing it on his skin causing burns to his legs and body. Mother has grabbed the 9 y.o. by the back of the head and rammed child into the concrete wall. Caller heard a thud. Severity of harm high due to mother's inappropriate disciplining actions. [LEB_case file]*

The case file reviews showed that reports of physical abuse were most common for ethnic minorities (see Table 3.1). This is contrary to the finding by Thoburn *et al.* (2005) who report that in the UK, physical abuse is more prevalent among Anglo families than Black families. In this Australian data, both cultural and acculturative reasons most explain its prevalence: (i) the use of physical discipline is culturally normal, acceptable and of value (especially in the area of scholastic achievement to enhance the family name); and (ii) due to lack of awareness of child protection systems (combined with a fear of authorities), disclosures of physical abuse are greater.

Thus, assessment of physical abuse and engagement with ethnic minority families in culturally appropriate ways is particularly pertinent; not all ethnic minorities who use physical discipline are physically abusive, and ethnic minorities should not feel culturally disempowered or disrespected by the imposition of absolutist criteria. The role of reporting biases should also not be overlooked when making sense of prevalence data.

Cultural acceptability of physical discipline in collectivist cultures

The trend among ethnic minorities is that the use of physical discipline is normal, acceptable and/or of value (Marie *et al.*, 2009; Pelczarski and Kemp, 2006; Qiao and Chan, 2005; Fontes, 2002; Trogan *et al.*, 2001):

> *Child: In Vietnam, they don't care if you hit your children as long as they don't die. [VIE_case file]*

> *Mother not willing to change discipline techniques, "I am sorry, you are not talking to a druggie, I am well educated". Father says mum has a traditional Lebanese attitude when it comes to disciplining the children, i.e. that physical force is appropriate. [LEB_case file]*

> *According to Vietnamese culture, children always obey and respect parents. Even if they punish [or] discipline them, wrong or right, they absolutely respect and obey the parents' orders. According to Australian culture, you call us 'abusing' or 'violent, domestically'. But according to Vietnamese culture, that's a normal, typical thing – if they [children] do something wrong, they [parents] beat you. [FAM_Vietnamese]*

> *In Burundian culture, if a child does something wrong, we are allowed to punish them physically and no one will accuse you of doing nothing. And if a child is a bit old, like 14 and above, you can take him to police, and police can also beat children. In a culture for millions, that's how I have been raised, which means we raise our children depending on how we've been raised. That creates a big problem for us in Australia. Our children are taught that your parents are not allowed to punish you physically, and if that happen, they should call police. When police comes, they arrest you or take your children away. That's a huge contrast to our culture. [FAM_Burundian]*

Importantly, not all ethnic minorities see the use of physical discipline as acceptable, highlighting the importance of acknowledging intra-group variation and not negatively stereotyping ethnic minority families:

> *Carer (maternal aunt) expressed she utilises 'time out' or take away privileges and/or talk through the issues. "No child abuse here whatsoever, did not believe in that method at all". [LEB_case file]*

NF told NM he does not like children being hit because when he was a child he was also hit by his parents and he knows how it feels. NF stated he is aware of the impact the children may have on hitting. [LEB_case file]

Also, the belief that physical discipline is an acceptable way to raise children is not exclusive to ethnic minorities; it may also occur among Indigenous and Anglo families. As one Anglo caseworker said:

There's nothing wrong with physical punishment. I think the cane is good. Now case managers are very young, and just want to cover their ass. They don't know. They just come out of university, which is teaching them what the one standard ideal should be. [CW_ANON]

Education and physical discipline in collectivist cultures

The cultural acceptability of physical discipline in collectivist cultures occurs for a range of reasons. Sometimes, it is seen as 'character-building, vital to the development of strength and endurance' (Hesketh *et al.*, 2000, p. 871). Sometimes, it is seen as necessary for maintaining the family hierarchy:

Pacific Islander parents in the western suburbs of Sydney commonly report they need to use what is regarded to be coercive strategies, such as shouting, yelling and smacking to get children to comply with their requests. This approach results in families coming to the attention of child protection agencies, which comes as a shock to parents who see themselves as caring for their children, by providing them with the discipline required to live in a hierarchical society in which respect and obedience are key values.

(Crisante, 2005, p. 3)

And sometimes it is related to the collectivist value for education. The educational achievement of children is the means by which families can increase their name and standing in the community. Failure to secure a highly respected position in the community may lead to social isolation, avoidance of which is important, as (visibly different) migrants are likely to experience social exclusion, racism or discrimination from the mainstream. It may also be that ethnic minorities have high academic expectations as a pathway to securing economic stability:

NM frustrated with her son for playing play station, rather than study. "You will make me sick if you don't do your work". Her frustration stemmed from her high hopes for his future. [VIE_case file]

As much is riding on the educational success of their children, parents may use physical punishment as a justifiable reason to ensure the child's scholarly achievement:

A lot of Asian cases were discipline-related to their not studying. [CW_Anglo]

Child stated father got angry whilst doing homework. Pushed his head down hard on the table and hit him on the back of the head. The abuse seems to occur around tutoring and homework, when he struggles to get things right. Younger brother (only in Year 1) sometimes made to stay up till 11pm to finish homework. Reporter [teacher] concerned father is using inappropriate physical discipline and due to high expectations academically [and] unrealistic pressure in regards to homework. Mum is aware of this violence and sometimes asks dad to hit them. [VIE_case file]

Example of good practice 4.1 –
Culturally respectful and helpful intervention from school

Kids said step-dad is really happy when they receive awards at school, so caller has sent them home with a principal award. [VIE_case file]

In one report, it said:

The parents and DG [Director General] shall consult with the principal about the appropriate amount of academic activities outside of school hours, and the parents shall not pressure the child to engage in a level of study outside that advised. Note: This excludes Tuesday Chinese classes. The parents agree to use their best endeavours to facilitate a sporting activity for child to attend after school or on a weekend. Note: At the current time, child's school work is not a child protection concern, though one of the issues that lead to verbal and physical abuse resulting in child's [prior] removal was his school work. [CHN_case file]

This case is an example of poor practice because there is assimilationist intervention from the school and the child protection system. Hypothetically, if an Anglo family were living in China, the father physically assaulted the child because they did not meet his expectations for sporting achievement and a Chinese caseworker intervened by suggesting the child take up extra-curricular maths tutoring, the intervention would unlikely be seen as culturally appropriate by the Anglo family; the outcomes desired by the father who values sporting excellence will not likely be attained by academic excellence instead. Such an intervention could also be construed by the family as a form of assimilation. Thus, it would be more appropriate for the Chinese caseworker to acknowledge the cultural value for sporting achievement among Anglos, explain the harmful effects of physically punishing the child for not meeting their expectations about it and introduce other forms of parenting that do not cause harm to replace the harmful parenting behaviour (e.g. time-out). By making a hypothetical point in reverse, it can be shown that this intervention would be a sign of cultural awareness and respect for cultural differences in parenting.

Additionally, in this case, the child was removed for two years from their parents. This is an example of over-intervention, given that physical assault due to academic expectations was the only reported issue for this case. By comparison, there was one Anglo case file from the same regional Community Service Centre (CSC), predominantly Anglo, as the aforementioned Chinese case file. The Anglo child was reported to be experiencing a whole range of abuses and neglect, such as 'emotional and verbal abuse', exposure to 'father seeing prostitutes' and 'mother injecting speed', displaying behavioural issues such as 'abusing people in the street' and attending court 'for bashing her mother'. Yet, the case plan for this child was to keep the child with the family, when removal may have arguably been considered more appropriate. Thus, failure to understand cultural needs may have contributed to this 'over-policing'.

Lack of awareness of child protection law among ethnic minorities

Some ethnic minorities may be aware that physical punishment is against the law:

> *It is hard here because the law is different but you have to do what the law tells you to. [CHN_case file]*

> *Uncle stated he would like to discipline the child "the Samoan way", however he believes he cannot as this entails "belting him" and he understands this is against the law. [PAC_case file]*

However, as ethnic minorities usually have less awareness of institutional systems like child protection, they may not be aware that it is illegal:

> *We say, 'it's not right to hit your child'. That's the broad thing. But there is a difference. Anglo families understand that's wrong and they'll do it. Families from a different culture, might not understand that the legal system here is quite different. [CW_NESB]*

Low awareness of the role of child protection authorities, combined with a fear of authorities, means that ethnic minorities may more freely disclose maltreatment without realising the consequences of doing so:

> *A lot of the time, CALD families will not educate themselves about child protection until DoCS becomes involved with their family, and that's a problem. 'Do you understand the role of DoCS?' 'No' 'Do you understand there's child protection laws?' 'What are they?' 'Do you understand you can't hit your child around the head?' 'Why not[?]' Then it gets to a point where you say, 'Do you understand your child can be removed from your*

care for these reasons?' People in other communities know that's the risk when DoCS get involved. They are aware of [the] legislation and that these organisations exist, but CALD communities aren't aware that we can do that until we actually tell them. So a lot of the time, they're giving really honest answers. [They] give you enough information to remove the child because they don't understand the process. If they know you're going to take their kid, they're going to alter them [their responses], just like Anglo and Aboriginal families do – that are clearly aware of DoCS' role. [CW_NESB]

Thus, lack of awareness of child protection systems can put ethnic minorities at risk of increased, inequitable and disproportionate exposure to the child protection system; that is, prevalence of physical abuse is partly greater for ethnic minorities due to reporting biases. Caseworkers should clearly clarify their role and statutory power as early as possible when engaging with ethnic minority families.

Culturally appropriate analysis: it's in the details

Since physical discipline is of value in some communities, there is a point at which physical discipline can become physical abuse or that physical discipline is mistaken as physical abuse, and it is critical that child protection authorities identify that point correctly or it becomes a threat to the safety of children and their culture:

Most caseworkers struggle with physical discipline being ok in some ethnic groups and child protection legislation [saying], to some level, that can be physical abuse. 'At what point does it become abuse?' Communities struggle with that. At one community information session, the African leader was saying, 'in our culture, we hit our kids when they do something wrong. Why is it we come here and all of a sudden we are treated as criminals for that?' There needs to be more emphasis on the fact that physical discipline happens in various ethnic communities [but] it becomes something against the law when, 'is it an open or closed hand?', 'is it above the head, below the waist?', 'is there an injury?', 'an open or closed wound?', 'yes, this is a common practice in that ethnic group but it's not a common practice to the point where a child's ended up with extensive injuries'. [Both] communities and caseworkers need to be provided with the skills to make the decision between physical discipline and physical abuse. [CW_NESB]

Previous research seems to suggest that child protection workers do tend to converge in their assessments of physical abuse, regardless of the child's ethnicity (Jent *et al.*, 2011). However, it is still critical to find the point that balances child safety, respect for cultural diversity and the observation of legal standards. This can be difficult when the legislation permits physical discipline, but the preferred policy is 'zero tolerance':

You have cultures that believe in smacking [but] DoCS says no to smacking at all, which is interesting. Legally, you are allowed to smack your child from the torso down without an implement, [but] it's difficult telling a family that 'legally you can, but we don't advise you to, we don't want you to'. [CW_NESB]

When you speak to families who come from countries where that has been the norm, the everyday practice, and it's not against the law there, how are we translating that back with our laws as 'zero tolerance'? We need to take different cultures into account. It doesn't necessarily mean that family doesn't love their child. [CW_NESB]

Hahm and Guterman (2001) also note that 'strong resistance (in Korean cultures) remains to the labelling of any physical discipline, including severe physical discipline, as *child abuse*' (p. 170). They call for recognition of cross-cultural understandings of abuse that must be within the context of recognising 'cultural autonomy' (p. 171).

It is even a challenge for some ethnic minority caseworkers, who are institutionally required to prioritise the child's safety over cultural knowledge:

A lot of the time, CALD caseworkers will go into families and see that the parents are actually trying to do the right thing, but may still be forced to remove or something along those lines. That's a real struggle for CALD caseworkers. [CW_NESB]

Culturally appropriate engagement: respectful education to promote insight

Since ethnic minorities are unlikely to be aware of child protection laws, it is critical that caseworkers educate families about them. However, the *way* in which this is done is important: they should not feel belittled or inferior for their lack of knowledge. That is, respectful and non-judgemental engagement is required, so that professional and institutional power is not abused:

If you are able to say to your client, 'I understand that education is really important in your culture. I understand that it means status, income, so many things that are important in that culture. I understand that is the problem that is causing the physical abuse', [that's respectful]. [CW_NESB]

This is especially important because even established migrant groups may not be aware of child protection laws:

People who came out 30 years ago have held onto their culture, even though their culture has changed. If Australians held onto their culture from 30 years ago, we'd still be using the cane. [CW_ANON]

It is important for caseworkers to acknowledge that within 'the migrant context', ethnic minorities hold onto parenting norms and behaviours (including harmful ones), because their culture, at the time of migration, is acting as 'an anchor' and any attempt to change this may be perceived or experienced as a fear of psychological and/or cultural loss. Such fear may cause the family to defend the harmful parenting, justifying culture over the law:

> *NF informed caseworkers that he can hit his son when he likes and that Australian laws are wrong and he should be allowed to hit child when he is naughty. [VIE_case file]*

To ensure ethnic minorities do not feel that their *whole* culture is under threat, caseworkers need to emphasise that it is only the specific, harmful behaviour they are required to dispel; they are not being asked to change their cultural values or norms, but simply change one part of their behaviour that will allow them to be law-abiding citizens who do not cause harm to their children. Arguably, cultural change may occur across second and third generations, and if so, such change would be generated from within members of the cultural groups and thus be empowering.

Education can promote insight into the harmful effects of excessive physical discipline, and is seen as a culturally appropriate 'first step' of engagement:

> *Harm was substantiated, however harm in the future cannot be substantiated at this point as the grandmother is in agreeance with the Dept's expectations re: physical discipline. [PAC_case file]*

> *NF acknowledged the impact on the children and the emotional scars that could remain. Both parents appeared regretful for their actions and genuinely concerned and are keen to repair the damage and ensure their children's safety. [CHN_case file]*

> *There was a Chinese family [with] 5 or 6 reports [of physical abuse]. Everyone agreed this is too much. Clearly, this father does not know it is not right and he's not going to change. You can tell when a parent really does acknowledge, 'this was wrong', 'that time my wife shouldn't have been doing that'. They have some insight into the effect that may have had on their children. It doesn't have to be a great insight, just something, it's better than none really. You can see they are 'workable'; you can work with those people. When a parent has nothing, doesn't want to acknowledge or take responsibility for anything they have done, then you know it's just not going to work. Where people put the responsibility back onto you, 'you never referred us to anywhere, you never helped us when we wanted to, we always did it ourselves', not taking into account that they've hit their child about 7 times with a belt leaving welt marks [and] exposing [them] to ongoing domestic violence. We throw that word [insight] around. I don't think we stop and think how much*

*our decision-making [is] based on the parent's level of insight into the needs
of the kid. [CW_NESB]*

It is important to note, however, that the goal of promoting insight is not easily
achieved:

*Mother reported to be affectionate but lacks insight into the effects of physical
abuse. [CHN_case file]*

*Mother does not acknowledge the violence in her use of punishment. Her
intent was to discipline child. [CHN_case file]*

*NF: "Australian law is different to Chinese law but if you do something
against the law it is not a crime". This evidences NF's complete refusal to
understand how he was harming his child. [CHN_case file]*

*Violent discipline from father. Both parents maintained that physical
discipline is useful in teaching children to behave appropriately. They regard
this as discipline and differentiate it from abuse. [CHN_case file]*

The difficulty of achieving insight may not just be related to the doggedness of
cultural values but to other stressors for families; if there are many, the harmful
effects of physical abuse may be minimised by families:

*If refugees [have] been able to survive, and women who have been raped,
they will have very little understanding of, 'oh, I cannot hit my child'.
[CW_NESB]*

Thus, realistic expectations are required:

*We try not to set our parents up to fail, as well as keeping in mind that the
children are our main concern. [CW_Anglo]*

Overall, respectful education to promote insight requires patience with all
minorities – newly arrived and established. As an example:

It is critical workers exhibit cultural sensitivity toward the parental use of
corporal punishment and understand the bitter feelings and resentment
[Korean] parents [in the USA] have when being accused of child
maltreatment. Parental defensiveness can often lead to potentially hostile
and adversarial encounters. To achieve effective service outcomes, workers
are advised to offer parent education regarding the negative effects of
corporal punishment and appropriate methods of discipline that would be
helpful and effective.

(Chang *et al.*, 2006, p. 889)

Arguably, respectful education to promote insight is required for all families:

> *It's easy to say, 'this is what child protection is and this is what risk is', because we've got legislation to back us up. The way it is communicated and explained is probably where we fall down. Saying to a family, 'you can't hit your child' when that's all they know, that's all they've done, that could be not even a CALD family, we don't explain very well about what the impact is of hitting a child. [CW_Anglo]*

Examples of good practice 4.2 –
Educating parents

Letter sent to NM outlining the Dept's concerns with her method of discipline. Several brochures were included: NGO support, alternative to hitting children, children and discipline, parenting tips. [PAC_case file]

Given there may be a lack of understanding/insight into Australian laws, it is recommended that the mother be educated around what constitutes acceptable discipline and what is not. Alternative disciplining methods to be explored with mum. Referrals to appropriate supports and services is recommended. [LEB_case file]

One way to deliver this education is through the use of ethnically matched caseworkers. This could help address the issue that families perceive their culture under threat and in turn defend maladaptive parenting behaviours:

> *Physical discipline commonly described as a cultural thing, however this is more of an excuse. Mandarin-speaking CW explained that it is not acceptable in Australia under any circumstances and it's necessary the parents understand this. [CHN_case file]*

Another way, at a more systematic level, would be to deliver this education through preventative outreach programs (see also Chapter 11):

> *We are running a few information sessions about the Department to African[1] communities in the area, and that is slowly, effectively, building our relationship with them. If we continue that on a regular basis, and become more active in those communities, we will have a very appropriate partnership. [CW_NESB]*

This kind of relationship-building is a particularly useful strategy because ethnic minorities, by virtue of having lower awareness of child protection matters combined with a fear of authorities, are generally more compliant than Anglo and Indigenous families:

[CALD families] are more likely to be compliant with us because of that fear of the legal system and the government. So we are able to say, 'you need to do this to make sure your child stays in your care'. Whereas Anglo families already have this idea of us being 'the bad guys' [so] they are sometimes more defiant. [CW_NESB]

When it comes to Indigenous families, the whole Stolen Generation, they are part of the Australian history. Indigenous families might think, 'you're taking our children away. Aren't you just doing the same thing as what happened in history?' Whereas a CALD family wouldn't understand that whole thing, so they wouldn't have as much negativity towards us. [CW_NESB]

Importantly, such a preventative 'outreach' program would not only help educate families about the harmful effects of excessive physical discipline, but also help offset the systematic entry of ethnic minorities into the child protection system due to their uninformed disclosures.

**Example of good practice 4.3 –
Not going straight to removal**

A lot of the time, we've told them they are not allowed to do it [physical abuse], and it is a one-off. [It] never comes back again. It is the fact that this community is not aware of the laws here, so they've done it. [But] there are other cases where it comes back, and comes back, and you get to the point where, 'ok, it's not good enough, this child is not going to be protected there, regardless of culture, regardless of belief. We have to take more severe intervention'. We need to be aware that there is a borderline for all clients regardless of their race [or] cultural background. If the child's not safe, we need to bring that child out of there and make sure they are. Our focus is the child, regardless of what background they are from, what their beliefs [and] values are. [CW_NESB]

Physical abuse and religion

Physical discipline/abuse may also be tied in with religious factors. Religion is cultural in the sense that normative characteristics 'belonging' or inherent to the group explain the occurrence of abuse. It is different to collective culture in which abuse is normalised for reasons that protect the family name and hierarchy. Thus, in the way that some individuals may justify the use of physical punishment in the name of culture despite the law, some individuals may justify the use of physical punishment in the name of religion despite the law. Importantly, fundamentalist individuals from any religion may pose similar issues in the child protection context.

Case Study 4.1 – Physical abuse and religion

NF [church minister]: I don't want my children involved in criminal behaviour, that's why I discipline diligently. Read from bible "blows that wound, cleanse away evil". It is an obligation from God to look after my kids. It's my responsibility to discipline the children. I use the belt on all my kids so that they will be good citizens of Australia.

CW: Common law not to use implements.

NF: You're assuming everyone knows the law.

CW: I'm just telling you. No implement which leaves mark, no physical force.

NF: The bible guides me. It allows me. You have your own man-made laws, but the only law I believe in is the bible. If God thinks what I am doing is wrong, God will punish me.
[PAC_case file]

Key points

- Physical abuse is the most common type of maltreatment reported for ethnic minority children.
  - o Part of its frequency can be explained by the widespread cultural acceptability of physical discipline (to build character and preserve the family name and hierarchy, especially through the child's scholastic achievement).
  - o Part of its frequency can also be explained by the higher disclosures of maltreatment among ethnic minorities because of their fear of authority and lower awareness of the role and statutory power of child protection workers to remove children.
- Distinguishing between physical discipline and physical abuse is critical for accurately assessing child safety and protecting cultural safety.
  - o The use of physical discipline is not exclusive to ethnic minorities, not all ethnic minorities use physical discipline and not all ethnic minorities who use physical discipline are physically abusive.
  - o Negative stereotypes about the prevalence of physical abuse among ethnic minorities can risk physical discipline being mislabelled as physical abuse in specific cases, inappropriately bringing children and families into the child protection system.

- Culturally appropriate engagement with ethnic minorities involves respect for cultures to be different in parenting values and practices, education to help promote insight into the harmful effects of excessive physical discipline and of alternative parenting techniques, and awareness of 'the migrant context' in which harmful behaviours are held onto even among established groups.
  - Intervention for parents who justify the use of physical punishment in the name of culture or religion should focus only on the harmful behaviour, not the cultural values that give rise to it. Families may be then less likely to defend harmful behaviours for fear that intervention is in relation to their whole culture or religion.
- The effectiveness of education to promote insight will be affected by the deep-seatedness of cultural values – generally and as migrants with fear of loss of their culture – and the presence of multiple other stressors that can lead to minimisation of risk of harm.

Recommendations for practice

- ✓ Consult with a 'multicultural caseworker' on a case-by-case basis to ensure analysis of when physical discipline has become physical abuse is accurate.
- ✓ Clearly tell ethnic minorities at the outset that caseworkers have the legal power and authority to remove children based on their disclosures.
- ✓ Explain the difference between lawful and unlawful use of physical discipline (e.g. open-handed strike, use of implements, etc.).
- ✓ If resources permit, allocate two caseworkers:
  - One who is ethnically matched to explain the law and help reduce the chances of parents defending harmful behaviours because of perceived threat to culture.
  - Another who is not ethnically matched to help offset the risk that the family perceives the ethnically matched caseworker as a cultural 'sell-out' or the fear that the non-matched caseworker may be culturally unaware or racist.
- ✓ Develop and implement preventative outreach programs that educate ethnic minorities of child protection laws, especially regarding excessive physical discipline and abuse.

Sexual abuse

Reports of sexual risk of harm, assault or abuse were reported in all case files:

Risk of sexual harm. Exposure to sexual acts. [ABR_case file]

NMs de facto was "sexing him with his penis". [ABR_case file]

Healed anal fissure suggestive of sexual assault. Blood on toilet paper. [VIE_ case file]

Sibling – inappropriate sexualised behaviour towards subject child.² Child said sibling told his mother a story about a Chinese ghost possessing him to explain his behaviour [rubs on top of her till he orgasms]. [CHN_case file]

Substantiated sexual abuse perpetrated by step-father. Allegations include touching child on the breast, indecent assault and digital penetration. Child does not wish to reside in the family home as she was raped there two years ago. NM does not appear to have insight into the danger of the situation. Child recently miscarried. Not the first, father was her step-father. There is a current AVO excluding step-father from the premises. [ABR_case file]

The nature of sexual abuse is the same across cultures, indicating that cultural factors do not need to be considered when substantiating it:

If sexual abuse is substantiated, then in most cultures that's pretty clear. I've not come across one where that's been vague. [CW_NESB]

However, the prevalence of sexual abuse does seem to vary across cultures: the case file reviews showed that reports of sexual abuse are highest among Aboriginal and Anglo families. This, however, does not mean that they are more sexually abusive than ethnic minority families, because sexual abuse is not condoned in any culture; there is no component of it that is seen as culturally normal, acceptable or of value (different to physical abuse in which there is a cultural component). As Fontes *et al.* (2001) say, all ethnic groups believe that child sexual abuse is a major concern.

Thus, the cross-cultural differences in prevalence are more likely to be due to a range of reporting biases. The 'culture of silence' that normally surrounds sexual abuse – that it is difficult for victims to make disclosures because of the unequal power relationships between adult and child and associated stigma (Fontes and Plummer, 2010; O'Leary *et al.*, 2010) – interacts with the cultural need to maintain family privacy and protect the family name for collectivist ethnic minorities. It also interacts with cultural norms 'in minority cultures, where matters of sex and sexuality are not discussed' (Chand and Thoburn, 2006, p. 374) and where family honour is typically important (Gilligan and Akhtar, 2006). In other words, various types of 'cultures' make it seem that sexual abuse is significantly less prevalent in ethnic minority groups, and explains the rate of *reporting* across cultures but not the true *prevalence* of abuse across cultures:

Mother's level of protectiveness is questionable. It appears she has coached child not to disclose [sexual abuse]. Interpreter said "child said 'I didn't tell them anything, I said no to everything'". [VIE_case file]

Child describes that it is difficult to attend her own faith church as in her culture she needs to be introduced to the Mormon church through a family member and her family are not willing to do this given she has made [sexual abuse] allegations about her step-father and the church believes the step-father is innocent. [PAC_case file]

In Middle Eastern culture and Islam, talking about sex is just so wrong. You don't ever do it. To be able to disclose that 'someone touched me in that way' – if it was a parent, an uncle, someone's friend – I could just imagine the difficulty the family would go through, the embarrassment. I've read stories where the most horrible things have happened to the child and no one has suspected a thing. [CW_NESB]

Cultural norms on emotional expressiveness are also discussed in the literature. According to Cohan (2010), 'Apollonian' cultures (e.g. Chinese, UK) are differentiated from 'Dionysian' cultures (e.g. Mediterranean countries, USA) in that in Dionysian cultures it is culturally acceptable and valued to display a larger range of emotional expression. Futa *et al.* (2001) also note that:

Middle position virtue is when the individual blends with others in society to maintain harmony, conformity and inconspicuousness. This differs from the European American culture which generally rewards individual creativity, assertiveness and initiative. The perpetration of abuse does not conform to the rules of society and allegations of sexual abuse are conspicuous and violate the middle-position virtue. These values can either decrease the incidence of sexual abuse among Asian American families compared to other American families, or serve to mask their reporting.

(p. 195)

There is also a higher level of awareness of sexual abuse in mainstream Western cultures which may additionally contribute to the higher rate of reporting among Anglo families:

In Anglo culture, sometimes we go overboard. We see a male with a little girl and automatically think, 'what's going on?' They are more suspicious because we are so aware of it [sexual abuse]. [CW_NESB]

Thus, the 'culture of silence' that typically surrounds sexual abuse is exacerbated in collectivist groups due to norms on protecting family privacy and family name, norms on the expression of sexual matters and lower awareness of sexual abuse. These all serve to create vast cross-cultural differences in reports of sexual abuse.

Perhaps these differences will change across generations. Indeed, Katerndahl *et al.* (2005) found more of a correlation between acculturation level and reporting of child sexual abuse than between ethnicity and reporting:

[It] depends what you see as important to those children that have come from another culture but are living here. What implication does that have for them when they grow up and decide that their upbringing is not the way they want to go? They've been exposed to another culture, another way, 'I don't have to put up with being sexually assaulted every night by my brother because my dad thinks it's ok'. [CW_Anglo]

Importantly, there is a racist element to the disclosure of sexual abuse among ethnic minorities that further complicates the aforementioned reporting biases. As Wilson (1993) puts it, 'when a white child is sexually abused, they think they are bad and dirty. When a black child is abused, she thinks she is bad, dirty and an affront to the race. She thinks, too of the message it will send to white society if she tells' (cited in Jackson, 2010, p. 7). The matter of sexual abuse and culture is deeply complex, and should be treated as such; simple attributions to the apparent prevalence statistics are unethical.

Case Study 4.2 – Culture, acculturation and sexual abuse

Earlier reports in case file

NM said there are cultural differences, and kissing and hugging in public is seen as inappropriate in her culture. She will speak with her husband and set some boundaries, and if she has any future concerns she will alert authorities. She was also thinking about sending child back to China. Child has stated that her mother is overprotective and doesn't understand Australian culture. Her step-father has made no inappropriate comments and has not touched her in an inappropriate manner. She has no fears for her safety.

Later reports in case file

NM has observed her husband touching the subject child on the breasts and has kissed her passionately. The POI [person of interest] has stated that he won't have sex with her until she is older but will continue to kiss and hug her and play with her breasts. Child is not uncomfortable around step-father. Child dismissed allegations of sexual abuse. Counsellor at NGO explained appropriate and inappropriate kissing. Mother described that the husband kisses the child in the same manner he would kiss the mother (romantic); the husband said to the mother "because Chinese women can't kiss properly I am teaching her how to kiss properly". Step-father has indicated his intention to have sexual intercourse with the child when she turns 16 and then consents. Mother viewed this is a good thing as the husband was waiting for the child to get older. [CHN_case file]

Key points

- Sexual abuse occurs in all cultural groups.
- Culture does not explain the nature of sexual abuse, because the nature of the perpetration is the same across cultures.
- Culture does not explain the prevalence of sexual abuse, only the rate of reporting, because no culture condones sexual abuse.
- Families from collectivist cultures can perpetuate the 'culture of silence' that typically surrounds sexual abuse if it is more interested in preserving the family name than protecting the child's safety; in turning 'a blind eye' it condones it and fails to protect children.
- Apollonian cultures – that value moderate expression of emotion – will also use 'moderate' language in such sensitive matters.

Emotional abuse

The most significant characteristic of emotional abuse is verbal abuse (e.g. yelling, swearing, threatening, criticising/chastising, etc.). It can lead to fear of the abusing parent and/or fear of going home. Emotional abuse is also often tied in with other forms of harm such as physical abuse and risk factors such as domestic violence and mental ill-health of parents:

Children shouted and sworn at. [PAC_case file]

Threatened to withhold love from child/criticised the child. [ABR_case file]

Involving child in her problems is considered emotionally abusive. [VIE_ case file]

Mother verbally abusive, causing children to have low self-esteem. [ANG_ case file]

Verbal abuse "I'll make you cry blood". Psychological harm due to instability and transferred parental stress. [LEB_case file]

Risk of emotional and physical harm high given the serious DV. Father threatened mother with a knife in front of the child. [CHN_case file]

Concerning psychological harm as child has stated he is very scared of his father and will only see him if a caseworker is present. [VIE_case file]

Father verbally abuses children because they are overweight and makes comments like "you are fat and disgusting". Risk of psychological harm. [LEB_case file]

"She hits you because you eat too slowly?" "Yes, she says I'm stupid and ugly and I eat too slowly". Threatened with knife. Could kill her at any time. [VIE_case file]

Being threatened to be sent back to live in China for not behaving well. Such chastisement is real and scary for child, whose 6 year old sibling resides in China. [CHN_case file]

Child disclosed to teacher's aide that no one at home loves him. He has been told to pack up and go. Mother doesn't call him by name, calls him "the little mongrel". Emotional abuse. Persistent caregiver hostility. Mother blames him for his sister's death. Mother once said to child in front of school principal "I wish it was you who died in the accident". [PAC_case file]

The case file reviews showed that emotional abuse was the most common secondary type of maltreatment reported for almost all families, regardless of their cultural background (see Table 3.1). However, the ways in which culture may be related to this prevalent form of maltreatment requires more research to enhance good practice with ethnic minorities; at this stage, little sophisticated and nuanced understanding is known about this relationship. Glaser (2002) also says that 'professionals find difficulty in recognising and operationally defining emotional abuse, and experience uncertainty about proving it legally' (p. 697):

When it comes to emotional abuse, you get to this grey area. How do we explain that verbal and emotional abuse is not appropriate to someone who comes from a culture [where] it's alright to talk like that to your child because it's discipline? Then there's religion. In Islam, a woman should always cover themselves, a girl doesn't go outside the home, shouldn't talk to boys. To us, it might be emotional abuse. You have to be careful. Stepping over the line, saying 'your religion is wrong', you can't say that. [CW_NESB]

Emotional abuse [is] very difficult. Caseworkers may not be able to source where certain behaviours are coming from. That's partly a lack of knowledge in being able to identify emotional abuse in comparison to cultural practices. [For example], children from various cultures will not look someone older than them in the face. A child will have his head down the whole time you are talking to them and caseworkers will either 1. perceive, 'this kid's not even listening' or 2. 'this kid's upset or emotionally abused or has no attachment or bonding'. These assumptions are made on the cultural practice. That can be difficult. You see that on a practical level a lot. [CW_NESB]

Key points

- Emotional abuse is the most common secondary type of abuse or neglect across cultural groups.
- The most significant characteristic of emotional abuse is verbal abuse.
- Emotional abuse often co-occurs with physical harm.
- Significant risk factors of emotional abuse are exposure to domestic violence and mental ill-health of parents.
- More research is required on how culture and emotional abuse are related; cultural and/or religious practices may be incorrectly used as evidence for emotional abuse.

Inadequate supervision

Inadequate supervision is marked by abandonment of children (including giving children to child protection systems), leaving children alone, with strangers or in the care of older parentified siblings, and lack of concern from parents on the child's whereabouts or their safety:

Caller wants to relinquish her rights as a parent. [ABR_case file]

Current whereabouts of natural parents unknown. [ABR_case file]

NM leaves children with anyone including strangers. [ABR_case file]

Child being left to care for himself while parents went to China. [CHN_case file]

Child left in car alone at night for at least 45 minutes in an RSL car park. [VIE_case file]

Children frequently seen without supervision and are known to be continually roaming around the streets including at night. [PAC_case file]

Child seen playing by himself in McDonalds and has fallen asleep. Police brought child home and was concerned since all adults had fallen asleep and no one had gone looking for the child. [CHN_case file]

Child stated she was home alone last night with her two brothers. Mother went out at 9pm. Child thinks mother went to the community club. Child went to bed and is not sure what time the mother came home. [VIE_case file]

Of all the characteristics of inadequate supervision, leaving children alone or in the care of older parentified siblings, are related to culture. The first is because children are typically allowed to be left alone in the country of origin (i.e. it is culturally normal) and so differences in child protection laws lead to the labelling of neglect. The second is because older children from collectivistic cultures are socialised to be responsible for family affairs at earlier ages than their individualistic counterparts (i.e. it protects the collectivist value for the family unit), but parentified children are seen as evidence of neglect from parents.

Leaving children alone

Ethnic minority parents may leave their children unsupervised because they did so in their country of origin:

> *In my country, schools not very close, but kids go alone. I go alone when I six years old. [FAM_Lebanese]*

> *Family migrated 12 months ago. Mother stated that in China parents are allowed to leave the children unsupervised. [CHN_case file]*

> *NF inquired what age it would be appropriate for child to be left home alone. Advised it was not recommended till he was at least in high school. NF was surprised with this answer and advised that in China child would be considered old enough to look after himself. [CHN_case file]*

In addition to child protection laws being different, leaving children alone may also be because communities (e.g. neighbours, extended family, etc.) typically play a significant role in child-rearing (see Chapter 1), reducing the need for primary carers to be substantially present:

> *Parents not looking after them – it's a cultural thing. It might be a neighbour from the same culture looking after the kids. The parents not being that primary caregiver gets reported [as] inadequate supervision. [CW_Anglo]*

For the same reason, parents in ethnic minority cultures may rather leave their children unsupervised and alone than let them stay with others who are not from the same cultural group and/or involved in the care of the child:

> *Parents [who work late hours and are thus unable to supervise child after school] have not permitted child to stay with friend after school. [CHN_case file]*

Leaving children alone may also be because of cultural beliefs:

> The Chinese saying, 'a child comes from nature and can be raised by nature' refers to the belief that 'nature' is an adequate custodian of a child's basic needs. Thus, phenomenon such as unattended children at home and neglect of

a child's emotional needs may be seen as normal from a traditional Chinese perspective, but would constitute child abuse according to Western norms.

(Lau et al., 1999, p. 1171)

**Example of good practice 4.4 –
Giving parents 'the benefit of the doubt'**

The times where the Korean parents aren't home – instead of waiting to meet the parents and look hard at finding them first, before a decision was made, to find that they were actually very loving, committed and capable people. It is a cultural issue. They didn't know the rules of this country. They have never had child protection. Needing to continue to think outside the square with that. [CW_Anglo]

Thus, to ensure these culturally normal behaviours are not mislabelled as neglect in the Western country, it is important to re-examine the assessment criteria. This is because inadequate supervision due to other risk factors of child maltreatment (e.g. poverty, domestic violence, alcohol or other drug issues, etc.) is different to inadequate supervision due to cultural misunderstandings about what is seen to be 'neglectful parenting':

Child absent from school due to looking after younger siblings. [PAC_case file]

Children not properly supervised by natural parents. NF works from 2–10pm so is unable to provide any supervision. [PAC_case file]

Mother stated that children were left alone because she has to go to work. Mother [also] explained that usually the father is with the children but due to the AVO this was impossible. [CHN_case file]

He missed the last weeks of school prior to the school holidays due to the family's homelessness however it appeared that NM needed his support to manage the younger three children. [LEB_case file]

It is also important to respectfully educate ethnic minority parents of the dangers of leaving children unsupervised, which may be different in the country of origin. This can help make their risk perception more culturally appropriate and thus increase insight into the harmful effects of leaving children alone in the new country:

She trusts her children and has explained to them what to do and what not to touch. The dangers of leaving the children alone was [then] explained to the mother. [CHN_case file]

Father spoken to in relation to lack of supervision and impact on children. Children are vulnerable to harm when left unsupervised due to their young age (6 and 9 yrs) and did not know how to get in contact with parents. Parents agreed not to leave children unsupervised. [CHN_case file]

I worked with [an African mother]. She left her children unsupervised for hours and hours, but that's what she did back home. She couldn't understand why it was an issue for us. I don't know how you get around that, because there's potential for risk in terms of children accessing the stove or whatever and that's really basic. How it's communicated, ultimately, that's going to make the difference. [CW_Anglo]

As with all matters, individual variation will occur. Thus, not all parents will demonstrate insight:

Parent's attitude towards inadequate supervision is that in China children are left home alone, despite being informed Australia operates differently. Caller stated child (9 y.o.) is responsible for running a bath for himself after school, which heightens his risk of burning. [CHN_case file]

Child left at home unsupervised until his parents or brother return home from work, late at night. He walks himself to and from school on a regular basis. Like any 8 y.o., he visits friends in the neighbourhood while left on his own, leaving the home unlocked and exposing himself to harm in the community. Both parents show limited insight into the concerns around leaving child unsupervised. [CHN_case file]

The school are struggling to get the mother to pick up the youngest from school and expects the other children to be in charge of this responsibility. The principal will speak to the mother again about how dangerous it is to have children walking down the street on their own. School have tried a number of strategies but mother continues to neglect her child and the school needs DoCS intervention. [LEB_case file]

For the same reason, not all families will need to be educated on the new risks:

Some items, especially electricity, gases, we don't have them in Sudan. If you learn how to use them, and prevent children not to get into [them], that's the most important thing. In Sudan, we were staying in the bushes, so you can protect your child from snakes, reptiles, fire, all these kind of things. We don't have those here now. [FAM_Sudanese]

Leaving children in the care of older parentified siblings

Children from collective cultures are usually socialised to be responsible for and contribute to the family collective at ages younger than their individualistic counterparts. This could lead to labels of parentification and thus evidence of neglect from primary carers:

> *Mother is not home when children come home from school. Oldest daughter (13 y.o.) cooks for the children when they come home from school. [LEB_ case file]*

> *In Australia, we have the belief that children under 16 shouldn't be left alone, or the sibling shouldn't be taking care of the younger sibling. So in some cases [CALD] parents have been charged with neglect even though that's normal in their culture. [CW_NESB]*

In Western and individualistic cultures, children are reared to become independent, responsible and self-sufficient adults, as these characteristics are of value. However, childhood is also seen as a 'golden time' that should not be 'stolen' by the responsibilities of adulthood. Thus, when some of the parenting responsibilities are given to the eldest child in collectivist families and they have greater family responsibilities than their age-matched individualistic counterparts, this may be seen as risk of harm to that child and labelled as 'parentification' rather than being labelled as socialised to be 'responsible' for family affairs, which is probably the intention of the ethnic minority parent. Thus, it is vital that caseworkers are not quick to judge or label culturally normative practices in collective cultures as harmful and accuse parents of neglecting their children as if there were mal-intent in their 'inadequate supervision'. To do so, is to demonstrate the problems with an absolutist approach to child welfare, as if one universal standard is applicable to all children regardless of their cultural context:

> *Neglect is an area we could do more work, on what's culturally appropriate. In Australia, age is the primary factor that makes you a child [but] in a lot of other cultures, responsibility level is what makes you a child or an adult. We can't just say, 'It's neglect, it's inadequate supervision, because a 12 year old is left caring for a four year old'. It can't be blanket rules. [CW_NESB]*

Example of good practice 4.5 –
Cultural awareness regarding 'parentified' responsibilities of children

I like [my] caseworker. She understands I'm Lebanese, [so] the way we raise our kids, you always expect something from my eldest girl. [FAM_Lebanese]

Perhaps most importantly, both culture and neglect may be occurring, in which case the relative contribution of each factor would need to be accurately considered:

Concerns children are caring for themselves. [PAC_case file]

Cultural issues with parents around supervision. Natural parents are aware they are not to leave child alone even for a short period. Harm assessed as concerning given the child is only 7 y.o. and was left home alone unwell for three days. [CHN_case file]

The children are vulnerable to risk of psychological harm given they are being parentified and providing care for their youngest cousin (5 y.o.) beyond their responsibility. Mother has been told that this needs to cease and that she needs to prepare her child for school. Mother does not seem to understand that it is her responsibility, not the children. [LEB_case file]

Key points

- Inadequate supervision is a type of neglect marked by abandonment of children (including giving children to child protection system), leaving children alone, with strangers or older parentified siblings, and lack of concern for the child's whereabouts or their safety.
- Inadequate supervision occurs in all cultural groups, but is related to cultural factors for collectivist/ethnic minority families when children are left alone or in the care of older parentified siblings.
- Leaving children alone may occur if this was normal in the country of origin – due to differences in child protection law, sharing child-rearing with extended family and neighbours and/or cultural beliefs about 'nature' being a sufficient guardian.
- Leaving children in the care of older parentified siblings is normal in collectivist cultures, because the child's level and sense of responsibility to the family collective is of value; age is comparatively less important.
- Level of insight may vary between families, with some showing an understanding of the dangers associated with leaving children unsupervised and others not. Risk perception may depend on individuals, awareness of child protection laws and number of other stressors within the family.

Recommendations for practice

✓ Consult with a 'multicultural caseworker' to ensure culture is appropriately considered and thus avoid inaccurate assessments or false accusations of neglect; blanket rules about the age-appropriateness of leaving children unsupervised should not be used.

✓ Respectfully educate ethnic minorities to promote insight into the harmful effects of leaving children alone, without disempowering their right to be culturally different.

Neglect of basic needs

In Chapter 3, neglect of basic needs and educational neglect were separated in analyses upon advice from caseworkers in a small validation/pilot study. However, since educational neglect was not found to be the primary type of maltreatment in any of the case files, it questions the validity of having it as a separate category. Thus, in this chapter, educational neglect has been incorporated into one type of 'neglect of basic needs'.

This is consistent with Tufford *et al.* (2015), who report that 'neglect can take many forms such as failing to provide adequate food, clothing, shelter, supervision, medical care, emotional care or education' (p. 230). It is also consistent with Seth and Raman (2014), who identify four main types of neglect: *physical* (e.g. hygiene, clothing, food and shelter), *medical* (e.g. nonadherence, noncompliance, delay or failure to obtain health care), *emotional* (e.g. failure to provide love and affection[3]) and *educational/developmental*.

Thus, when neglect was found in the case files, reports pertained to educational, nutritional, medical and housing[4] neglect. Importantly, these four types of neglect of basic needs are strongly associated with one another, so children experiencing one type are likely to be experiencing others as well:

Does not have home-made dinners, she buys take away. [ANG_case file]

Extremely skinny and malnourished. Basic physical needs not being met. [VIE_case file]

Irregular school attendance. Children asking for food from neighbours. [ABR_case file]

Inadequate furniture and bedding. Inadequate nutrition also reported. [PAC_case file]

200 spiders on the kitchen ceiling. Past non-school attendance. [ABR_case file]

Medical neglect. Mother left hospital without a medical discharge and/or medication. [LEB_case file]

Concerns in relation to the children's hygiene. Youngest child regularly arrives late to school in a dirty shirt and has no food in her bag. [LEB_case file]

Both children overweight – lots of maccas [McDonalds] boxes lying around house – children may not have their nutritional needs being met. [ANG_case file]

Reporter said house was disgusting. There was a very strong smell of urine, phlegm in the ashtrays, house did not appear to be cleaned for months. There was food scraps and rubbish, broken windows and holes in the walls and grime all over the kitchen cupboards. Reporter's colleague believed that children should be removed from the house. [ANG_case file]

Overall, neglect of basic needs is independent of culture; no group sees it as normal, acceptable or of value, nor as protecting the collectivist value for the family unit. Thus, neglect is due to other generalist risk factors such as domestic violence and alcohol or other drug issues, but especially poverty (Slack *et al.*, 2004).

Culture may only be relevant in assessment of children's development where culturally *irrelevant* criteria are used to judge families, highlighting that it is important caseworkers do not mislabel culturally normative practices as possible or actual neglect of children:

DoCS reported in interview with NM and NF that a negative aspect of the children's development was that they didn't know how to use spoons. NM stated they used their hands to eat and that "that's our way". Possibly related to cultural practices. [PAC_case file]

Key points

- Neglect of basic needs includes educational, nutritional, medical and housing neglect.
- These four types of neglect of basic needs are strongly associated, so children tend to experience a few of them rather than one in isolation.
- Culture is not related to neglect of basic needs; it occurs because of other generalist risk factors of maltreatment.

Notes

1 African families are a newly emerging group in Australia.
2 Rapoza *et al.* (2010) call for more research on sibling abuse.
3 Withholding affection is seen as 'emotional abuse', and different to 'emotional neglect' or failure to provide affection. Here, emotional neglect has not been deemed a type of 'neglect of basic needs'.
4 'Housing neglect' has been differentiated in this study from 'housing issues', the latter referring to current, fear or threat of homelessness (see Chapter 5), and the former referring to inadequate provision of household items (e.g. bedding).

5 Common risk factors of maltreatment

Are domestic violence, alcohol and other drug issues, mental health issues in the carer, housing issues and financial issues related to culture?

Prevalence of common risk factors across cultural groups

Some of the most common risk factors of child maltreatment (especially emotional abuse) are domestic violence, alcohol and other drug issues, mental health issues in the carer, housing issues and financial issues. For example, emotional abuse was the primary type of maltreatment in 1/20 (5 per cent) Chinese, 4/18 (22.2 per cent) Lebanese, 1/20 (5 per cent) Pacific Islander, 6/20 (30 per cent) Vietnamese, 3/20 (15 per cent) Aboriginal and 3/20 (15 per cent) Anglo case files, and in all cases the cause was attributed to exposure to domestic violence, alcohol and other drug abuse and diagnosed and undiagnosed mental health issues in the natural mother. Data on these five risk factors were scoped for in the case files. Importantly, they are all 'generalist' risk factors (rather than 'cultural' risk factors) because they occur in all families. Having said that, they interact with cultural factors for ethnic minorities (see each section below).

The data in Table 5.1 shows that, not including financial issues, domestic violence is the most common risk factor of child maltreatment for families from all six cultural groups, alcohol and other drug issues are the next most common risk factor and mental health issues in the carer are another significant risk factor. Financial issues were not counted in this study because so many of the cases in the case file reviews had received financial assistance (see Chapter 2). That such

Table 5.1 Generalist issues reported by cultural group

	N	DV (%)	AOD (%)	MH issues in carer (%)	Housing issues (%)
Chinese	19	9 (47.4)	2 (10.5)	6 (31.6)	1 (5.3)
Lebanese	19[1]	12 (63.2)	6 (31.6)	9 (47.4)	6 (31.6)
Pacific Is	16[2]	11 (68.8)	6 (37.5)	6 (37.5)	4 (25)
Vietnamese	20	11 (55)	6 (30)	6 (30)	1 (5)
Aboriginal	20	16 (80)	16 (80)	7 (35)	4 (15)
Anglo	20	13 (65)	12 (60)	8 (40)	3 (15)
Total	114	72 (63.2)	48 (42.1)	42 (36.8)	19 (16.7)

Note: DV – domestic violence; AOD – alcohol and other drugs; MH – mental health

assistance was provided and commonplace indicates that financial issues are a generalist issue common to groups of all cultural backgrounds in the child protection system.

Domestic violence

The impact of domestic violence on children varies from exposure to being harmed while intervening during an incident of domestic violence. Cases may or may not include threats of or actual physical violence during verbal arguments. Mostly, the perpetrator is male, but damage to the victim is equally severe:

> *She hits me in front of the children. I told her not to do it. I try retraining myself. We men suffer, can't say anything. [CHN_case file]*

> *Children exposed to ongoing and extensive DV between the natural parents. Witnessing NFs continual threats to kill NM and the children. [ANG_case file]*

Domestic violence is a generalist issue – it occurs in all families regardless of their cultural background. However, it interacts with cultural factors for ethnic minorities, most especially the pressure to keep family matters private, protect family cohesion (or 'togetherness') and save face:

> *Mother refused to provide a statement to police and get photos taken of her injuries. [LEB_case file]*

> *Pressure from family to drop assault charges and AVO against father. [VIE_ case file]*

> *NF indicated he did not normally discuss the family's problems as this [DV] was a private matter. [CHN_case file]*

> *NM holds fears for her safety due to previous physical abuse by her husband that she was afraid to report as it would bring shame to the family. [LEB_ case file]*

> *NF indicating he wants to keep his family together. After some discussion, NF agreed to supports/referrals, originally hesitant due to shame/embarrassment. NF: "Can we keep confidential, can spark more problems. Wouldn't want matter exposed". [CHN_case file]*

Thus, in cases of domestic violence, the pressure to keep family matters private may mean that family members experience tension between two of their own conflicting needs – to seek help on the one hand, and protect the family name and keep the family together on the other. This is especially true for ethnic minority women. 'Because of the power structure of many Western legal and social institutions as Eurocentric and androcentric, many ethnic minority women do not want to bring attention to their problems for fear of stigmatising their family and communities' (Kanuha, 1994, cited in Yick, 2007, p. 279). Similarly, Wurtzburg (2000) says, 'with regard to shame, women bear the greater proportion of social and family blame when a male partner is violent' (p. 22). One (male) interviewee also said:

> *In Iraq, the famous point in our culture is – they don't go [to] the police, because it's a shame for the woman [to] bring the police for the husband.*

Fear of the perpetrating spouse for disclosing abuse to authorities may also prevent victims of domestic violence from seeking help. As Giglio (1997) says, 'in cultures where men are considered superior to women, they may fear reprimand if they tell of abuse at home' (p. 5). Importantly, fear of disclosing abuse to authorities is not exclusive to ethnic minority families, but may be heightened in families with traditional gender roles.

The cultural value for family cohesion particularly plays out in the lack of enforcement of Apprehended Violence Orders (AVOs):

> *There is an AVO in place though the father has indicated he will lie for the mother to keep the family together. [CHN_case file]*

> *Mother taken out AVO on father but does not abide by Family Law Court (FLC) order – mother allows father to have contact during dinner time with the children. [LEB_case file]*

Caseworkers need to acknowledge and report the difficulty for ethnic minority women of enforcing AVOs:

> *AVO protecting mother and children from father, [but] mother not being protective, not enforcing AVO. [LEB_case file]*

> *The mother is not accepting any responsibility for keeping the children safe. She has indicated she will leave the father in the event of another domestic incident, however she has said this in the past and not followed through. [LEB_case file]*

While the assessments are accurate in terms of child safety, they fail to demonstrate awareness of the difficulty for ethnic minority women to enforce AVOs because doing so threatens family cohesion, paramount in collectivist cultures. As it is, 'parents who are usually the main support for children in providing nurturance and protection may not be able to do so when they are exposed to, or are victims of, (domestic) violence themselves' (Osofsky, 2003, p. 162). Selwyn and Wijedesa (2011) also say that domestic violence 'prevents many mothers from being able to protect their children' (p. 282). Victims of domestic violence, regardless of their cultural background, also find it difficult to leave for a host of psychological reasons, and so both personal and cultural factors need to be taken into account when addressing domestic violence with ethnic minorities. Thus, failing to understand, acknowledge, document and/or attempt to meet this conflict for ethnic minority women suffering domestic violence is an example of poor practice.

Moreover, ethnic minority women may perceive that they *are* protecting their children by keeping the family together: by protecting the family's name and their place in the community, the children reap the benefits of family cohesion and community belonging and aid. Thus, 'failing to protect children' can mean different things to a caseworker and an ethnic minority woman. Arguably, ethnic minority women suffering domestic violence say they will leave the harmful situation but only because they feel pressured to say so, and thus, why they do not actually enact it. Perhaps if they were given empathy for what may be lost, culturally speaking, she could then leave the harmful situation. The empathy may allow her to perceive the threat of safety to her children in the way the caseworker perceives it, rather than downplaying or denying it. It may also help counteract any fears the mother is having that the caseworker has come with 'Western beliefs' about choice and freedom and independence that she may not have (perceived or actual):

> *NM getting calls from mother and father-in-law saying 'we'll fix it between us'. NM said "no it's too late, I'm protecting my daughter". NM saw the counsellor who made her realise that she needs to protect her children. [LEB_case file]*

In short, the collectivist values for family name and family cohesion may make reports of domestic violence lower for ethnic minority groups, reduced by these culturally determined reporting biases, but that reports of domestic violence in this data set are quite high for all groups indicates that cultural norms about keeping family matters private are superseded when police are involved, and cases of domestic violence are formally recorded. Thus, in relation to the child protection system, culture is most related to domestic violence in the lack of enforcement of AVOs.

Example of good practice 5.1 –
Culturally appropriate analysis and engagement regarding domestic violence

Children exposed to verbal/physical DV. Father yelling [and] choking mother. Father not charged, as mother did not want to give any information. Child afraid for mother's safety [and] scared she will get into trouble for telling [teacher]. NM understands that DV is impacting the children but has no plans to change the situation. NM hopes that one day NF will change.

> *NM unwilling to get AVO as she does not want to create hate between them. Action through DoCS home visit and phone calls, and providing links to external, culturally appropriate professional supports and services. NM has been sent pamphlets in Vietnamese about how DV can impact on children and services she can contact if needed. Child and sibling at risk of further harm without effective intervention, due to their presence in the home and the possible inability of the mother to ensure protective behaviours due to being a victim of violence herself. Further assessment warranted. [VIE_case file]*

Alcohol and other drug issues

Alcohol and other drug issues are another generalist issue that can bring families of all cultural backgrounds into the child protection system:

> *Inadequate nutrition as parents are spending all their money on AOD. [ANG_case file]*

> *Most [families] come in because of the primary reason of drug and alcohol, [then] you've got the secondary reason; because they are affected by a substance they are involved in DV or don't have the ability to parent. It's not a CALD issue, it's a lifestyle [issue]. [CW_NESB]*

Substances include alcohol, cannabis, heroin, Valium, morphine, cocaine, ice, speed and (meth-)amphetamines. In some instances, caseworkers need cultural knowledge to be aware of less commonly used substances:

> *Fijian families threw me a bit. You can't smell pot [or] see any beer bottles around. What the hell is going on? It's not adding up. You need to know what their culture uses to get off their face. [If] you don't know anything about 'kava', then you don't know what to look for. [CW_Anglo]*

Alcohol and other drug issues were noticeably higher in Aboriginal and then Anglo cases, and hardly an issue for families of Chinese background (see Table 5.1). Thus, culture is related to the prevalence of alcohol and other drug issues, in that in some groups, the use of (at least) alcohol is culturally normal and acceptable:

> *Not so much drug and alcohol issues [in this area] cos of the large Muslim community. [CW_NESB]*

In speaking of Vietnamese families, one caseworker noted that there were differences between 'eras' of families migrating to Australia after the war. This kind of contextual information is helpful for caseworkers:

Drug and alcohol [is] a problem in Vietnam. Those that came soon after the war and became refugees tend to do well, be law-abiding citizens, but those who lived in Vietnam for a long time after the war, got brought up in a society that was a very difficult period and people immersed into [drug] problems. They've brought with them a lot of those attitudes into Australia. A lot of [Vietnamese] clients on our system mostly relate to drugs. [CW_NESB]

Mental health issues in the carer

Mental health issues in the carer affect all families, and so this is another generalist risk factor of children being maltreated and entering the child protection system:

Child staying home from school. This may be to look after mother (in bed crying all day). [VIE_case file]

NM has untreated MH. Persons in the home are fearful of NM mood swings and her behaviours when she is behind closed doors. Both children said their mother is crazy. "She keeps on hitting me. Dad says it's cause she's mentally ill". After child was bitten by his mother, he picked up a metal sword with a pointy tip and charged at mother with it. [CHN_case file]

The two most common mental health issues of carers reported in the case files were depression and anxiety. Less commonly, bipolar disorder, borderline personality disorder, postnatal depression, schizoaffective disorder, schizophrenia, anger management issues and suicide attempts were also reported. These issues occurred most often in the natural mother.

In the same way that family privacy and saving face substantially interact with domestic violence, so too with mental health issues in the carer; the stigma associated with mental illness means that such issues are kept hidden from outsiders to protect the family name. Thus, parents are not likely to take up support services they would otherwise benefit from (see also Chapter 6), and will prefer to address such issues within the close family:

NM requires help with the children due to her MH, so the extended family help care for the children. Family is very supportive and protective. [VIE_case file]

Some ethnic minorities do access services, highlighting the importance of not stereotyping families:

I see a psychiatrist [because] it's nice to talk about it. You shouldn't keep it inside, cos then you get sick. [But] I'm different. In our culture, [if] you see a counsellor or a social worker or a psychiatrist, some [people] think you're sick. It's just their mind. I take depression pills. If I was in Egypt, [they would think] I'm mentally sick. But it's not something bad, we're just trying to look after ourselves. Some people are scared to talk [but] it's your right to talk about what you feel. We [are] living in Australia [now]. [And it's a] free country [so] you can say what you want, what you feel. [FAM_Egyptian]

As with all generalist issues, it is also important not to racialise them by, for example, overstating the role of culture or ethnicity:

I had this one extreme, complicated case. The other caseworker was trying to over-emphasise that they were Arabic and Lebanese [but] I believe it got a lot more to do with mental health issues [in the child]. He was in a refugee camp for about 9 or 10 years and was sexually abused while there. Now, at the age of 12, [his] actions [are] uncontrollable. The mother also has mental health issues. In that matter, it wasn't cultural at all. Anybody who has been through this circumstance would probably have that [challenging behaviours]. [CW_NESB]

It is also important not to racialise post-traumatic stress disorder (PTSD) for refugees, simply because it is prevalent in this group. That is, PTSD is a mental illness caused by exposure to trauma, not by being a refugee or an African (for example):

We've got a lot of reports with African people in regards to mental health issues. I don't want to stereotype [but] based on my experience, [when] African people came here, [they] already got mental health issues [from] back in their countries. [CW_NESB]

A lot of our clients are refugees or have come on humanitarian visas [so] it's not like they've just decided to come to Australia. Their history involves a different pattern, as opposed to people in the top section [of the Australian] system that have not had that exposure to extreme stress and trauma. [CW_Anglo]

In short, culture affects mental health issues in that they are usually kept hidden. Further, mental health issues should not be understood along racial/ethnic lines.

Housing issues

Housing issues are marked by current, fear of or threat of homelessness. They are a generalist issue because they occur in all families:

Mother will be homeless as of tomorrow. NM received another termination letter from the real estate agent and was told to go to a refuge. [LEB_case file]

> *Homelessness due to eviction. NM stated the children are distressed as they continually ask where they are going to live. Caller is about to be kicked out on the streets with her three children who are under 9 years old. [LEB_case file]*

Housing issues may be tied in with cultural factors in that some groups normatively have larger families than others. This may in turn be linked to inadequate shelter – a form of neglect – and bring children to the attention of child protection authorities. Where reported in the case files, the number of children in the household varied from one (Chinese) to 11 (Aboriginal), with an average of 3.6. The group with the largest average number of children in the household was Pacific Islander (M=5.2).

> *With African communities, we help them a lot with housing. Afghanistan as well – they are the ones who have large families. [CW_NESB]*

> *DoCS established the family as a priority. DoCS liaised with Department of Housing to arrange a new four-bedroom house. [PAC_case file]*

> *Some families come here with seven or eight children and they can't find proper housing, so they come into our [child protection system]. [They] become homeless. [CW_NESB]*

Housing issues may also be linked to culture in that migrant groups may not meet criteria to be eligible for housing assistance:

> *He phoned the Homeless line and was told they could assist himself and the child, but as his wife is a sponsored person and not a permanent resident, she could not be assisted, so he declined their assistance. NF said that they are homeless and that he has put in an application to Department of Housing for more long-term accommodation. [LEB_case file]*

Example of good practice 5.2 –
Cultural awareness regarding meeting housing needs

NGO CW said that DV victims from Middle Eastern background who reside in the [Western suburbs] area do not adjust well in the Eastern suburbs area. They tend to feel isolated and there is lack of culturally appropriate services. Suggested we consider a refuge in the [Western suburbs] area where she could have more supports. [LEB_case file]

Financial issues

Financial issues, including financial stress and hardship, occur in all families and so are a generalist issue:

> *Within this community, there are housing commission areas or particular suburbs that are really aware of welfare and DoCS, and you are going to have difficulty with those people regardless of where they are from. [CW_NESB]*

Culture may be related to financial issues in two ways. The first is through gambling. Gambling is a psychological addiction that can cause financial issues. It was identified in all the case files, but was notably prevalent among Vietnamese women. More research is required to tease out the roles of culture and gender:

> *Mother has severe gambling habit. [VIE_case file]*

> *"She has no money, she gambles it". Mother has gambled all their money and this happens quite often. [VIE_case file]*

Of more overarching importance, however, in regards to whether financial issues are related to culture, is that the way poverty affects risk of harm assessments may vary between Anglo and other caseworkers:

> *Australian caseworkers are more legalistic. They're not used to poverty. [CW_ANON]*

> *I went with [an] Anglo caseworker to a CALD family. She has three kids under five. Her house is a little messy, but the children have food in the fridge and are well cared for. To me, that is good. This caseworker recommended that this is neglect, and mum doesn't have parenting skills. We see things different, because of our background and experiences. We are more accepting, more flexible on making judgement on people. [The] consequences of those judgements are very harmful, damaging, to the family. The basic standards we expect from our clients are different. We come from poorer countries. People who have a higher standard, expect our clients to have a higher standard for their children. [CW_NESB]*

Thus, Western standards of poverty should be appropriately questioned with ethnic minorities from developing nations to ensure that risk of harm assessments are accurate. It taps into a bigger issue of exercising caution when comparing any two countries that differ greatly in affluence because, as Mildred and Plummer (2009) say, 'it is easy to fall into the errors of judging other societies by our own standards and assuming that our relative affluence means that we are more "advanced" and therefore culturally and morally superior to other nations' (p. 604).

Key points

- The five most common risk factors of child maltreatment (especially emotional abuse) are domestic violence, alcohol and other drug issues, mental health issues in the carer (especially the mother), housing issues and financial issues.
- These risk factors are generalist issues – they occur in all families regardless of cultural background. However, they interact with cultural factors.
- Domestic violence and culture:
  - It is difficult for ethnic minorities to hide domestic violence, as part of keeping family matters private, because it often comes to the attention of police.
  - As the cultural pressure to keep family matters private still operates, the true prevalence of domestic violence among ethnic minorities (and other groups) may still be hidden.
  - Ethnic minority women may want to seek protection and help from outside sources (like child protection authorities or family support services) but cannot because of cultural pressures to not shame the family.
  - The cultural pressure to keep families together (as part of collectivist cohesion) most commonly plays out through failure to enforce AVOs.
- Alcohol and other drugs, and culture:
  - Substances not known to or commonly used by the mainstream require cultural knowledge.
  - Cross-cultural differences in prevalence of substance abuse relate to cultural acceptability of their use (e.g. alcohol use normative among Aboriginal and Anglo families and not acceptable in Muslim families).
- Mental health and culture:
  - Pressure to keep mental illness private is heightened in collectivist families due to the associated stigma that would compromise the family name. Thus, support services are not commonly accessed.
  - Mental health issues are at risk of being racialised for ethnic minorities, for example, for refugees suffering PTSD; others also experience PTSD and refugees can suffer other mental health problems.
- Housing issues and culture:
  - Culture is related to housing issues when cultural groups tend to have larger families.
  - Culture may also be related to housing issues when migrant families do not meet eligibility criteria for housing assistance.
  - Culturally appropriate supports also need to be considered when meeting housing needs (e.g. refuge for Muslim women).

- Financial issues and culture:
  - Gambling can cause financial issues and seems common among Vietnamese women.
  - Western standards of poverty should not be used to understand ethnic minorities from poorer countries; it can compromise accuracy in risk of harm assessments.

Recommendations for practice

✓ Caseworkers should not racialise generalist issues; to do so pathologises culture and exemplifies racism. Consult with a 'multicultural caseworker' to avoid this.

✓ Acknowledge the difficulty for mothers in taking out or enforcing an AVO, as it breaches cultural norms about keeping the family together, but to iterate that such behaviours compromise the safety of the child.
  - Emphasise that all matters are kept confidential, except as required by law. As such, there is no reason to fear that the community would hear of the abuse and that there is no justifiable reason for them to 'suffer in silence'.
  - Remind the (mostly female) victim of domestic violence that its occurrence is cross-cultural – it happens to women from all cultures – and this is why extensive support strategies are available in the community to help them. This can help decrease any sense of isolation or loneliness they may feel.

Notes

1 Two Lebanese cases were of siblings in one family. As such, some of the descriptive quantitative analyses (where appropriate) are based on a sample size of 19 *different* case files, to account for intra-familial co-variation.

2 Three Pacific Islander cases were of children belonging to one family and another three cases were of children belonging to another family. As such, the 2x2 additional children in each family (n=4) have not been included in some of the descriptive quantitative analyses due to the high intra-familial co-variation. Thus, a total sample size of 16 different case files has been used for this group where appropriate.

6 Protective factors

Acknowledging strengths of families across cultures

In any risk of harm assessment both 'strengths' and 'needs' need to be carefully considered to help ensure accuracy (O'Neil, 2005; Cousins, 2005). It is in the child's best interest to see what the family does have rather than taking only 'deficit' eyes and seeing what they do not, and a strengths-based approach to practice helps promote resilience and personal agency (Maiter and Stalker, 2011):

> *Strengths – nil identified. [VIE_case file]*

> *Protective factors unknown. [VIE_case file]*

Ethnic minority families will have two types of strengths that should always be considered – those related to cultural factors and those that occur for all groups. This way, a thorough and holistic approach to assessment can be assured.

**Example of good practice 6.1 –
Thorough and holistic risk of harm assessments**

When we do [a] risk assessment, we do it holistically. We just don't look at one incident, we look at the whole family situation – whether it is going to be harmful or better for the child to be in that situation for a while. People who are living in that family who can be protective – if dad is abusive, is mum protective? The age and understanding of the child – if he or she knows she has to make a phone call [to] 000; [can they] protect themselves to a certain level? Service providers, neighbours, AVO are also other protectors [we look at]. [CW_NESB]

Cultural-related strengths are those that relate to collectivist features and/or cultural safety. Religion may also be a culturally related strength for some ethnic minorities, but it is distinguished from collectivist culture. Non-cultural strengths are protective factors not exclusive to ethnic minority (or Indigenous) families. Thus, they are not primarily about the preservation and safety of collectivist culture.

Cultural strengths

Valuing family cohesion

Since ethnic minorities usually come from collective cultures, one of their main strengths is valuing family cohesion or 'togetherness'. As Shalhoub-Kevorkin (2005) says, 'the strengths of the Arab family and society – mainly the social solidarity, economic assistance and psychological support of the collective (including the nuclear and extended family, neighbours, friends) – should not go unrecognised' (p. 1266):

> *In terms of strengths, the family appears to be close. [VIE_case file]*

Of course, protection of family togetherness as being in the child's best interest is not exclusive to collectivist families – a 'child-centred but family focused' approach to child welfare is necessary for good practice with all families – but it may be heightened for them because of the definitive value for it. As children are less seen as individual units in collectivist cultures, protecting children by prematurely removing them from family perpetrators of harm is a violation of how collectivist families see the safeguarding of children and undermines the value of this cultural belief, and therefore cultural safety (see also Chapter 2).

Thus, value for family cohesion should be fully taken into account when making assessments of the strengths of collectivist families, with acknowledgement that for cases that do not warrant removal, 'child protection' is best understood as keeping the family together. This takes a 'group' or social approach to child welfare, consistent with the values of collectivism. It also helps ensure that the safety of these cultural values is respected and preserved.

Supportive extended family and other supports

Another key culturally related strength of collectivist families is the presence of supportive extended family and community. This wide circle acts as a strength by keeping children at risk of harm within their kinship, important for later cultural and other developments related to sense of self:

> *NF: Large extended family that will "help out if we need it". [VIE_case file]*

> *Maternal grandmother came from Samoa to assist NM for a while with the children. [PAC_case file]*

> *In very remote areas in Asia, people function with nothing. Why is that? Because they have support. Everything is community-based. [CW_NESB]*

> *Mother was finally accepted by refuge [but] this may cause problems as mother is away from her Muslim community supports. [LEB_case file]*

Similar reports were commonplace in the Aboriginal case files. This is not surprising given that community-based values are also strong for this group. The strength of extended family and other community supports were less often reported in the Anglo case files, indicating that extra-familial sources of strength may not be sufficiently considered or reported on for this group; just because Anglo families are typically individualistic, it does not mean that the strength of supportive family and community is not relevant for them.

Importantly, although family and community support is a crucial strength for ethnic minorities, it may be withdrawn if the 'family name' is under threat due to involvement of child protection authorities. Thus, the need to respect family privacy needs to be strictly observed; if issues of confidentiality are not properly addressed in casework practice, the strength of family and community support may be lost.

Preserving culture

Activities that help preserve the culture of origin are also a source of strength for ethnic minorities because they help offset any feelings of displaced sense of belonging. They also protect cultural safety – the right of groups to 'be who they are' and co-exist with different others without judgement, disrespect and/or expectations to assimilate. This is critical because the cultures of non-mainstream (and Indigenous) groups are more under threat of loss in multicultural Western countries than the culture of the mainstream, and so the protection that those cultures offer in terms of belongingness need to be overtly and fully acknowledged:

Attends Arabic school. [LEB_case file]

Children participate in cultural events and learn traditional dance. [PAC_ case file]

Child respects people of her own Samoan culture as she feels a cultural connection to them. [PAC_case file]

Maternal uncle (carer) highlighted that in order for child to have a positive and stable life, it was important for him to grow up with his family, cultural and religious group. [PAC_case file]

Child reports to be enjoying these classes and has made many friends of Chinese background. Until restoration takes place, the Dept will be encouraging child to continue these sessions to maintain her cultural heritage and preserve already formed and established relationships with other children. [CHN_case file]

Willingness to engage with services

Resistance to use of preventative and other family support services in the local community is not exclusive to ethnic minorities but is lower for them for a range of reasons. Chand and Thoburn (2005) found that the use of social work services by South Asians in the UK was 'inhibited by a mixture of embarrassment, perceived stigma associated with seeking help from local authority services and parents being unaware of what was on offer' (p. 172). Hackett and Cahn (2004) also point out that some migrant families have 'reticence to access services (because of) less than optimal past treatment experiences or instances of negative interactions' (p. 17), which in turn could be related to perceptions of the service being culturally inappropriate:

> *[I] don't access services in the community. [I] don't trust them. These services seem strange. [FAM_Vietnamese]*

It may also be related to economic disadvantage in the country of origin. As Qiao and Chan (2005) say, 'the lack of attention to domestic violence and child maltreatment [in China] is also due to the scarcity of social services in the country' (p. 25):

> *If we started off with that opportunities [counselling services] back home, we would access it [in Australia]. [FAM_Sudanese]*

However, one of the main reasons is cultural: the pressure to protect the family's name and keep family matters private is so high in collectivist cultures that it even affects disclosure to the wider cultural community, so resistance to service uptake is understandably lower than in the mainstream. In keeping with this, Ward *et al.* (2005) found that urban and rural culturally and linguistically diverse (CALD) families' use of home and community services were proportionate to regional demographic profiles, suggesting that the effect of culture on service use extends above and beyond rurality.[1] Cultural barriers prohibit the full use of support services like parenting programmes or relationship counselling that could ease tension in the family that might otherwise lead to child maltreatment. These trends also flow across generations through modelling:

> *Child not actively wanting to engage [with services]. He is also aware that parents need to engage with services and is witnessing this not occurring, so may be modelled behaviour. [CHN_case file]*

Given the magnitude of cultural factors, it is an immense credit to an ethnic minority family when they do access such services; they will have had to breach severe cultural pressure to not share family matters with outsiders, including professionals. In other words, willingness to engage with services is a culturally related strength of ethnic minorities and this needs to be recognised and acknowledged by caseworkers:

I consented to Brighter Futures² cos I am open to extra help. Whatever is out there, I'm prepared to try cos I've got nothing to lose. I am so grateful and appreciate any help I can get. [FAM_Greek]

Parents now working in a more co-operative and open manner with the Department – mother accessing DV counselling and father has been seeing a counsellor re anger management and other issues. [PAC_case file]

Religion

Religion is a culturally related strength, different to the strengths that collectivism offers, and may be relevant for some groups:

NM: I asked child to be strong, to pray to God. I go to Samoan United Church. I explain my problem, they pray for me. It helps me. [PAC_case file]

Many members of the church around to help out (she is heavily pregnant). She is almost bored as no one will let her lift a finger. [PAC_case file]

Non-cultural strengths

Positive and engaging dispositions, insight and resilience in children

Characteristics of children that can be seen as strengths include a positive and engaging disposition, insight and resilience as a result of hardship. These should be properly considered and acknowledged:

Child presented as happy and outgoing who asked questions and responded well to questions asked. [CHN_case file]

People think refugees need all this help, but they are more resilient than people realise or give credit for [them]. [CW_ANON]

Child demonstrated a good understanding of why he is coming to counselling, "because dad hits us and stuff". [PAC_case file]

Secure attachment with parent/s

Even more important than characteristics of children that indicate (non-cultural) strength is secure attachment between child and parent/s (Wilkins, 2012; Krane *et al.*, 2010) when assessing risk of harm and making other decisions (e.g. possible restoration). Secure attachment is associated with positive parenting behaviours, good communication and expression of warmth:

Child has strong attachment and is affectionate with mother. [PAC_case file]

NM has good relationship with daughter and provides for her physical, developmental, psychological and emotional needs. [CHN_case file]

There appears to be a good relationship developing between child and his mother. This is demonstrated by the conversations child has with his mother – are not heated or about something he has done wrong. [ANG_case file]

However, secure attachment is not always marked by the same behaviours across cultures, and failure to understand cultural norms regarding parental affection and warmth is a barrier to good practice. For example, norms in emotional expression affect demonstration of secure attachment:

[At contact] they exchanged hellos, no hugs and kisses. [CHN_case file]

As people of Chinese background are generally modest in displays of affection, the caseworker's report required an additional qualifier such as '... however this behavioural exchange is not uncommon among families of Chinese background and so may not necessarily indicate a lack of parental warmth'. This would ensure the report was culturally appropriate.

Attachment manifesting differently across cultures can occur in a range of ways:

Child speaks about the mother not buying her things. Child feels that her mother does not care about her. [VIE_case file]

It's very difficult for people from CALD groups to express their feelings to their loved ones. They [tend to] show it through cooking [or] through buying something for you. We don't say [outright] "I love you". When caseworkers don't see any physical contacts, [they may think] "these children are unloved". We are very judgmental. We are not flexible. We don't factor in differences. We base [our practice on a] 'one-size-fits-all' in child protection. It doesn't work. [CW_NESB]

**Example of good practice 6.2 –
Considering attachment in risk of harm assessments**

[Italian] mum has mental health [and] drug issues [so child only] attended school every now and then. We were thinking about removing this child, thinking of her rights to be educated. But when you look at attachment, they are much attached. All her life, this child is always with mother. She doesn't have anybody [else]. She's happy there, they love each other, there is secure attachment between them. If you remove a child like that, it's going to do more harm. We ended up not removing her. Apart from her education, her medical needs are met, food, other things. Everything else [is] ok, [so] attachment is considered. [CW_NESB]

Acknowledging protective actions of children and parents

As equally important as it is to consider the attachment between child and parent/s, it is also important to acknowledge protective actions. These may be of children who engage in self-protective actions:

> *Child identified how to implement a safety plan if he ever is placed in danger at home. [PAC_case file]*

> *CW asked if she knew who to call if she ever felt threatened and she said DoCS and the police. [PAC_case file]*

However, it is more important to adequately acknowledge the protective actions of parents (which overlap with characteristics of secure attachment). These may include, for example, meeting basic needs under stressful circumstances, being supportive, contacting supports (e.g. counsellors, police, etc.), expressing warmth to and concern about children, implementing Apprehended Violence Orders (AVOs) and overcoming poor parenting behaviours that compromise children's well-being (e.g. drug use):

> *NM contacted police when the children absconded. [PAC_case file]*

> *Protective factors for [child] is that she attends school. [VIE_case file]*

> *Dept should recognise the strength it took for NM to overcome addiction. [ABR_case file]*

> *Carer stated that child's parents seemed very supportive of him whenever he saw them. [ABR_case file]*

> *NM demonstrated protective behaviours by speaking with counsellor and discussing her concerns. [CHN_case file]*

> *Mother presented as very concerned about her son, very capable of meeting his needs, and very loving. [VIE_case file]*

> *NM acknowledges her inappropriate behaviour and parenting of child and expresses her commitment to make changes. [CHN_case file]*

> *An AVO has been applied for against the NF. The NM stated she would abide by it and not invite the NF back into the household. [VIE_case file]*

> *NM continues to ensure that her children's basic needs are being met [despite DV]. They are attending school, after school activities, and are being taken to social events such as birthday parties and to school excursions. [LEB_case file]*

Key points

- To help ensure accuracy in risk of harm assessments, both strengths and needs need to be carefully considered; good assessments are thorough and holistic.
- Strengths for ethnic minorities may be cultural and non-cultural in nature.
- Cultural strengths relate to: (i) collectivism – valuing family cohesion, having supportive extended family and other community supports and willingness to engage with services; (ii) cultural safety – cultural preservation; and (iii) religion.
    - o   Willingness to engage with services is a particularly strong strength given how difficult it is to breach cultural norms of privacy.
- Non-cultural strengths occur in all families and include: (i) positive and engaging dispositions, insight and resilience in children; even more importantly, (ii) secure attachment between child and parent/s; and (iii) (self-)protective actions of children and parents.
    - o   Secure attachment is often associated with positive parenting behaviours, good communication and expression of warmth, but cross-cultural differences in norms on the expression of emotion need to be considered to ensure attachment is accurately assessed. Affection may not be demonstrated through overt affection and/or may be demonstrated through cooking or buying gifts.

Recommendations for practice

- ✓   Record all efforts to explore cultural *and* non-cultural strengths in case file notes so that neither are overlooked.
- ✓   Do not under-estimate the protective role of family cohesion for ethnic minorities when making risk of harm assessments.
- ✓   Adequately assure families of confidentiality so that the strength of supportive extended family and community is not withdrawn for fear of tarnishing the family name.
- ✓   Do not under-estimate the protective role of insight and resilience due to hardship in children when making risk of harm assessments.

Notes

1   Importantly, 'the literature on rural migration and ethnic communities has tended to occupy a marginal place in Australian social science' (Missingham *et al.*, 2006, p. 132). More research is required.
2   Brighter Futures (BF) is an early intervention program delivered by FaCS (then DoCS) for families at risk of entering the child protection system.

7 Working effectively with interpreters

It can be difficult working effectively in child protection matters when engaging with an ethnic minority family low in English proficiency:

> *We use interpreters and telephone interpreters and that's often difficult in itself. [CW_Anglo]*

> *For a Persian-speaking family we are currently working with, the only way we can communicate is via interpreters. That is extremely challenging and difficult. [CW_Anglo]*

Yet, it is a necessity. Inadequate interpreting services are 'detrimental to the needs of minority ethnic families, as well as the professionals involved' (Chand, 2005, p. 812). Humphreys *et al.* (1999) say 'the significance of the interpreter service, in the absence of a child protection system with workers representing the range of languages in a multicultural society, cannot be underestimated' (cited in Chand, 2005, p. 810):

> *[If] it was [the] ideal situation, we'd have someone that could speak every language in the office. [CW_Anglo]*

Importantly, 'the presence of an accent should not result in a presumption that a person requires translated materials or an interpreter' (Sawrikar *et al.*, 2008, p. 72), and caseworkers should engage with their client families in a respectful manner; 'raising the voice or verbal bombardment is usually unhelpful, as is constantly correcting the client's grammar' (Ely and Denney, 1987, cited in Chand, 2005, p. 817), for example. However, overall, the effective use of interpreters is most critical for accurately gauging a child's safety:

> *When you are trying to get what you mean in English, you may perceive that as 'wow, that mother was very negative', but maybe that's how they speak in their culture. [CW_NESB]*

Psychiatrist: I interviewed her in Cantonese. Her behaviour may appear inappropriate in the Australian setting but entirely appropriate in the Chinese culture. She just wanted to teach her son to be respectful to authority. She loves her son but her English is not good enough to convey her feelings. [CHN_case file]

Ethnically matched interpreters, in particular, can understand cultural nuances especially for explanations about the cause of maltreatment but also for understanding body language (Perry and Limb, 2004). For example, Owen and Farmer (1996) noted that 'in some Asian languages (in the UK) the words necessary for the description of sexual abuse do not exist, or are so rarely used that people would be shocked by their usage, [so] in many cases a balance had to be maintained between politeness and clarity' (cited in Chand, 2005, p. 811). Thom (2008) also notes that actions like head-nodding and smiling should not be assumed to indicate sufficient understanding:

They say 'yes', but it's 'yes' just to be polite. See, in our [Vietnamese] culture, first you try to please and if they don't know how to answer, they just have a smile. [CW_NESB]

Families may say 'yes', which the caseworker might interpret as confirmation they have understood what they just explained, whereas in fact it is simply an indication to keep going. [CW_NESB]

Chand (2005) also notes that:

The presence of an interpreter will often raise the anxiety levels of the social worker ... For the social workers, there may be a pressure to try and balance being concise with trying to convey the message appropriately. One obvious consequence in achieving this balance is that the attention of the social worker may become misdirected towards issues of language, instead of concerns about the child.

(p. 71)

Issues with interpreters

Inaccurate translation

Accuracy in translation was the only issue with interpreters cited by both family and caseworker interviewees, indicating that it is *the* key characteristic of good practice. As Križ and Skivenes (2010) note, loss of trust because of the lack of a common language can prohibit interactions necessary for establishing a good relationship, and in turn lead to loss of accurate assessments and access to services.

According to Baker *et al.* (1991), 'oral interpreting requires extremely good listening skills, immediate recall and an ability to convert meaning from one language to another on the spot' (cited in Chand, 2005, p. 808). Gonzalez (2005) also says that interpreters should maintain the same meaning, tone and register as the original message, without giving additional material:

> *There are interpreters that will interpret word for word, that will sit behind and be just a voice and not part of meanings. That works much better. [CW_Anglo]*

These skills form the basis of good interpreting, but are particularly important in child protection work. If, for example, the interpreter speaks on behalf of the individual or there is lack of accuracy where interpreters make significant omissions and mistakes (Chand, 2005), these significantly compromise the accuracy of risk of harm assessments:

> *Interpreter have to listen [to] you and explain everything as you say. Don't be twist way. [FAM_Ghanaian]*

> *Interpreting service good, but not always useful. Can't interpret exactly, 100%. That deeply emotion, that deeply feeling. [FAM_Vietnamese]*

> *I can't imagine how confronting it is for a family to have to trust that someone else is delivering their message to you. Word for word. The sentiment. [CW_Anglo]*

> *Sometimes the interpreter is difficult to understand. You don't know whether they have translated what you want to say. When they translated in English, are you perceiving the right way? There's that barrier when it comes to languages, where you say something but it means something different in another language. It's very hard. [CW_NESB]*

> *Interpreters are useful for the popular languages [but for] the new and emerging African communities, there is issues around getting access to interpreters that can speak English to a level that is required to interpret that conversation [and] what the legislation means when we are using our terms, without having a backwards and forwards conversation between them and the client and the caseworker just sitting there. [Sometimes] I have to jump in and say, 'Stop. Tell me what just happened. And ask me the questions'. [CW_NESB]*

Accuracy in translation is aided by rapport between interpreter and caseworker, because they help ensure that clarifications are sought:

> *Rapport between interpreter and caseworker very important. [CW_NESB]*

I find it very helpful when an interpreter says, 'the family really don't understand what you are talking about and this word isn't known in our language; can we try a different word[?]' [CW_Anglo]

However, rapport is best between interpreter and caseworker, rather than between interpreter and client family:

With a lot of new and emerging communities, as soon as they see each other there's an instant rapport, so the conversation, if you don't have enough skill as a caseworker to work out when that's got to be terminated, there can end up being a lot of issues. [CW_NESB]

Accuracy is also aided by the interpreter's skill level to ensure all voices are heard:

[We had] a young African boy involved in criminal activity [and] kicked out of home. We had a whole range of people in the room that did not speak a word of English and the interpreter on the phone. They were really good. Even though they weren't there, they were able to keep the conversation controlled, so when I was talking no one else was talking, when they were talking he would translate after each person spoke. It didn't feel like anyone was taking over or no one was not being heard. Everyone had a chance to speak. [CW_NESB]

In short, accuracy of translation depends on verbatim interpretation, that not all words and concepts translate in other languages, level of English in the interpreter, rapport between caseworker and interpreter, and interpreter's skill level to represent all voices.

Interpreters not sensitive to child protection issues

Another significant issue that arises with interpreters is when they are not sensitive to child protection issues:

Interpreters often get training on medical and general legal [but not] specific training on child protection. The manager and caseworkers should do the training, not people from Head Office, because we got knowledge [of the] barriers [of] working with CALD communities. Do role plays, scenarios from DV to drugs, child abuse, sexual abuse, everything, so these people can be exposed to working with [a] caseworker in child protection. [CW_NESB]

Providing training to interpreters in child protection matters can help avoid two serious risks to children and families. The first risk is that interpreters may intervene or advise in the child protection matter during the interview process:

> *Some interpreters will take on case management when they're not briefed properly. Especially with domestic violence. In some groups they will tend to be on the side of the man, especially if it's a male interpreter. They may say, 'you need to go back' [to the woman]. We need to be extremely careful in those situations. We may even need a pool of interpreters that specialise in certain issues. [CW_NESB]*

The second risk is that interpreters may make the session more about them, sometimes being related to their own life experiences:

> *We had removed a 15 year old girl because her family had threatened to kill her. We met with the family to talk about what happened and where to from here. When the mum was saying she can't believe her daughter had gone, it was really quite emotional. The interpreter started crying as well. It reinforced [the] mum, [and] escalated the situation. I signalled [to] her, 'It is not actually about you, it's about this mum who is obviously very upset about losing her daughter'. Often they are not [sensitive to child protection issues]. It's a training issue. We should be saying to the interpreter prior to walking into a meeting, 'This is what we are going to be discussing today' – a bit of briefing, so they have some idea [and] it's not a shock. Especially if we were talking about sexual abuse. Because you don't know their background either. You don't know their experience and how that might impact on them communicating with the family. I've [also] had interpreters tell you their life story and barely interpret what families are saying. [CW_Anglo]*

Thus, training and briefing interpreters is critical to good practice. Chand (2005) similarly notes there is a 'need to ensure interpreters are clear about their roles and responsibilities [and] can accurately and sensitively communicate with families' (p. 809).

Cultural biases in interpreters

It can be reasonably assumed that ethnically matched interpreters offer cultural awareness, understanding and/or empathy to the client family. However, this is not always the case. Cultural differences between two classes or religions within the same culture, for example, can produce biases and judgement in the interpreter (Korbin, 2002). In such cases, it may be useful to offer language-matched, but not ethnic-matched, interpreters (e.g. an Arabic-speaking Lebanese interpreter for an Arabic-speaking African client family). On the other hand, it may be important to have someone from the same culture, and not just the same language, because of regional conflicts (Giglio, 1997). Thus, whether language-matched or ethnic-matched interpreters are better depends on individual case needs.

Different dialects may be difficult to understand

Different dialects within the same language can be difficult for families to understand, and in turn, possibly compromise accurate assessments in child safety. Again, this issue highlights that there may be times for an ethnically matched, not just language-matched, interpreter:

> *The same cultural background is better, because Lebanese can be alright, but they having different accent in Arabic. For Southerners [Sudanese], they can't understand anything. [FAM_Sudanese]*

> *Two occasions I was provided with an Egyptian interpreter. She could not understand my Arabic. She could not convey what I really needed to do, so there was a language problem. [FAM_Jordanian]*

> *Different languages have different dialects. You could get a Hungarian interpreter who speaks the wrong dialect and they don't understand [so] you have to find someone who is available and does speak that dialect, and sometimes you can't. You sit on the phone in the lounge room and hope to God that they find someone. [CW_Anglo]*

Interpreters not gender-matched

The literature acknowledges the importance of gender-matching families and interpreters to observe cultural norms and/or in sensitive matters like domestic violence and sexual abuse (Chand, 2005). As Giglio (1997) puts it, 'it may be important to have women interpreters either because of religious beliefs or because the alleged perpetrator of the offence is male' (p. 6). Thom (2008) also says that 'certain religions may preclude female patients from having a male interpreter' (p. 29), so adherence to cultural norms is important. However, it is also important just for meeting personal preferences:

> *Got to be same gender. [FAM_Turkish]*

> *It's better for a woman to always have a woman, because sometimes you want to say something and you embarrassed to say it to a man. [FAM_Argentinian]*

Issues with families

Families refusing to use an interpreter

A significant issue that can arise with families is their refusal to use an interpreter when they would otherwise benefit from one:

Interpreter needed but refused, English not good but adequate. [VIE_case file]

Mother has indicated that an interpreter is not required but reporter [teacher] believes an interpreter would be beneficial for discussing complex matters. [VIE_case file]

No, never [use interpreter]. Yes, I don't 100% in English, maybe 50% English, but I don't need [interpreter]. When I need the interpreter, I can't speak English no more. [FAM_Lebanese]

We've got a Filipino mum at the moment. She speaks English but we weren't sure if she was really comprehending what we were telling her [so] we asked her about four or five times [if she] would feel more comfortable with an interpreter and she said, 'no, I'm fine, I understand'. 'Ok, the option is there if you need it, just let us know'. The majority of the time they say 'no'. [CW_NESB]

Thus, client families may refuse to use an interpreter, over-estimate their English comprehension and/or believe that the opportunity to practise their English is more important than accurately relaying information that pertains to the complex matter of assessments of child safety. While choice is important, it is also necessary that caseworkers explicitly emphasise the magnitude of their intervention, which ethnic minorities may not be aware of or understand (see Chapter 3). A basic level of English is not sufficient to understand technical information, especially when clients are stressed (Thom, 2008):

We also work with people that speak very good English, born Australian, [and] they don't even have the capacity to communicate with us, let alone the CALD groups. [CW_NESB]

There's a lot of terminology that you cannot directly translate in Arabic. You gotta walk around it and explain it that way. Like, there's no such thing as 'Department of Community Services' in Arabic. So you talk about how we're child protection, we're a government department, it's a building here, there's several of them ... [CW_NESB]

We have a very difficult language in child protection. I talked to a girl today, asking what 'sustainable', 'insight' [and] 'viable' mean. And she's an Aussie. If you're going to translate those words, you're going to have to use more words to make sense. We use very big words. That's the barriers we set. People don't understand us. [CW_NESB]

Example of good practice 7.1 –
Advising ethnic minorities to use an interpreter in court

CWs advised both parties to request an interpreter in order to explain the issues in court. [CHN_case file]

Families not wishing to use interpreters for fear of breach of confidentiality

As it is, there is loss of privacy for client families when using interpreters:

> *Not good [using interpreters]. Discussion between two is always better than between three. You feel your confidentiality, is feeling invasive. Two, you feel more comfortable. [FAM_Jordianian]*

However, this loss of privacy is exacerbated for families from collectivist cultures, who value keeping family matters private and protecting the family name; they may fear a breach of confidentiality from the interpreter. As Chand and Thoburn (2005) point out, 'despite valuing their ability to speak the same language and understand their culture and religion some (South Asian parents in the UK) experienced their support as intrusive and were concerned about possible lack of confidentiality' (p. 174):

> *They don't want their community to know what is going on with their family. [For] one Afghanistan client, I said I can organise an interpreter. She said 'no, no, I don't want them to know about us'. I said 'there are a lot of Afghans here. You might not know that person'. She said 'no'. This lady speaks about three languages [so] we organised an Arabic-speaking person not of [the] same culture. [CW_NESB]*

In such instances, families should be reassured that it is mandatory for all interpreters to keep matters confidential, except as required by law. Importantly, Chand (2005) notes that 'for some (South Asian) families (in the UK) it was important the interpreter was outside of the family's network or community ... (but) in a climate of rationed resources in local authorities, this raises the question of how likely it is that such a request will be met' (p. 810). Thus, resource limitations need to also be considered.

Families wishing to use their children as interpreters

Chand (2000) says, 'the use of children as an interpreter in child protection issues should be regarded as unethical and unprofessional' (p. 71). The child might not understand the exact nature of the problem being discussed or the subtleties of the language being used (Chand, 2005). Parents may not wish their children to know everything about their particular problems or it may be inappropriate for them to know (Chand, 2005). Finally, 'the child will have to make difficult choices about where his or her loyalties lie' (Chand, 2005, p. 815), which may then make the child be 'at the end of the parent's frustrations and anxiety from the process of disclosing highly sensitive or important information' (Giglio, 1997, p. 5):

> *[A] Pakistani woman brought her daughter to be the interpreter. We said, 'no, you can't do that'. We organised a telephone interpreter. Her daughter was there to witness the whole interview but we didn't actually utilise her as an interpreter. [CW_NESB]*

> *I don't think a lot of people are aware of all the power shifts that are involved in using children as interpreters. It affects the parent's ability to actually parent the child, when the child's in that powerful role to be able to transfer information and affect conversations. If people were aware of that, people would be less likely to do that. [CW_NESB]*

It can also lead to or exacerbate intergenerational conflict as a result of acculturative stress:

> *Child and mother experience conflict over cultural issues. Ongoing conflict re adolescent issues and the mother's reliance on child for help with the younger children and to interpret for her. [CHN_case file]*

Dominelli (1997) argues that 'exploitation of black children (as interpreters in the USA) is racist because it facilitates the continuation of inadequate services for black people' (cited in Chand, 2005, p. 815). Thus, when families 'initiate the use of children as interpreters, (they may be) responding to the inadequate interpreting facilities in the only way they know how' (Chand, 2005, pp. 815–16). Instead, they should be reminded they can bring a trusted confidante to act as an advocate for their needs and provide them support (Chand, 2005):

> *They're allowed to bring a support person. It can be anyone from [an] organisation, or relative or friend. It's usually a person they trust. [CW_NESB]*

Resource issues

Lack of (correct) interpreter available

It may not always be able to be addressed, at least in the short term, but it is still helpful to be aware that one significant issue when trying to work effectively with interpreters is the lack of an appropriate one. This resource issue is problematic because failing to give a voice to all family members with availability of an appropriate interpreter affects the caseworker's capacity to make accurate assessments of a child's safety. Chand (2005) also notes there is a 'need to ensure interpreters are available when required' (p. 809):

> *NF speaks limited English and there are currently no Tongan interpreters – messages passed through NM. [PAC_case file]*

> *Most of the time, they bring interpreters who speak Swahili because they don't find Kirundi interpreter. That's no good [for his wife] because his wife doesn't speak Swahili. [FAM_Burundian]*

> *There's barriers. Like Swahili, there's one interpreter in NSW, two Laos interpreters. Sometimes all you want to do is tick the boxes and make sure there's an interpreter there, but you cannot do that because you cannot get hold of these interpreters. [CW_NESB]*

Time intensity

Another significant resource issue is the time intensity involved in using interpreters. This can then cause caseworkers to avoid using them and in turn compromise accurate assessments of child safety:

> *I don't think we use them [interpreters] enough as we should. [CW_NESB]*

> *You have to allow double time when working with an interpreter. Sometimes we need to interview the parents twice, three times. We've got to interview all the people that we know. Caseworkers get reluctant to engage [an] interpreter because there are so many times you have to work with [them]. [So] we do less [and] shorter interviews. You don't get insight into the problems. [CW_NESB]*

> *We have an unlimited budget so that is lovely [but] everything takes twice as long if you use an interpreter. It's a difficult job as it is, but when you have to involve that [interpreters], it's a complicated process. The quality of the interpreters, depending on what the language is, luck, [all] that has a really big impact on your case load. You might get allocated one case but it is equivalent to two. [CW_Anglo]*

> *Counsellor: This process of counselling the child's mother and father is extremely difficult due to cultural differences and the need for an interpreter. Progress is painstakingly slow in that everything needs to be interpreted in both directions. NM's receptive English is much better than her expressive English, however everything goes through the interpreter, so what we would normally achieve in one hour would probably take three hours of counselling. [CHN_case file]*

That the use of an interpreter essentially doubles the caseload is important for case managers when allocating workloads. This is important for ensuring that full information is gathered about families with low English proficiency, and child safety assessments are not compromised. Chand (2005) has already cited insufficient time allowed for meetings as an example of poor practice. Thom (2008) also argues that while the use of interpreters during *all* stages of assessment and engagement 'appear[s] costly and unnecessary, it is a basic right for people to be able to access services' (p. 29).

Examples of good practice 7.2 –
Making allowance for the time intensity

It is important for caseworkers to have time and patience and respect [when working with ethnic minority families]. [CW_NESB]

CALD families just take a lot more time to work with than other families. Because of the concepts, you gotta do things twice over to get that message or information across. I don't know, maybe the second time round it just makes more sense. [CW_NESB]

Telephone interpreters

Thom (2008) asserts that for child protection matters, face-to-face interpreters should be mandatory because being able to see body language and facial expressions is necessary for establishing proper rapport. However, due to resource issues of face-to-face interpreters not always being available, telephone interpreters may be engaged instead. While it may be unavoidable, it is still important to acknowledge its associated limitations:

If using a telephone interpreter, my staff [are] like, 'who am I communicating with?' [CW_Anglo]

I am a trained interpreter myself [but] I find that with child protection, if you use a phone interpreter it's hard. It's hard enough with face-to-face. [CW_NESB]

Our telephone interpreter service [is] very impersonal. I know it's convenient and you can't always grab someone who speaks that language at the last minute [but] for a family you've been working with, and you know, they need an [face-to-face] interpreter. Don't have someone on the phone. It's rude. They understand body language and non-verbal signs and the intention behind what they are saying. [It's] heaps more beneficial. It's not just someone regurgitating in another language. Because [of] cultural differences, what we might see as offensive is not supposed to be taken that way at all. [CW_Anglo]

Other resource issues

Several other resource issues may arise, which may be difficult to avoid. These can include interpreters not arriving, conflicts of interest, lack of telephone coverage, interpreters not wanting to travel long distances and having to pay more to cover that distance, and having different interpreters on different occasions:

Sometimes you book [an interpreter] and they don't turn up. [CW_Anglo]

Sometimes you book [an interpreter] and they know the person so they can't go, which happens a lot with the Sudanese. [CW_Anglo]

What if you went to an area that has no telephone coverage? You get out there and they don't speak English. What are you going to do? We've got heaps of areas that don't have mobile phone service. [CW_Anglo]

I won't have a Persian-speaking interpreter come out to [suburb] [so] we have to arrange to meet the family in [another suburb] – it's just the distance. To pay someone extra to come out, that's been the biggest difficulty. [CW_Anglo]

If you book an interpreter it's not always the same one. That can be a problem when you try to build relationship of trust, 'this is a safe space', 'this is the interpreter'. It's like when you send another caseworker, it is a barrier. We want to form these relationships, but it's very hard when you're relying on external services that don't care who they send. [CW_Anglo]

Summary

Overall, the results indicate that (i) training caseworkers on how to work well with interpreters and (ii) training interpreters on how to work in child protection matters, is essential to assuring accuracy in translation and thus child safety. Chand (2005) also notes that 'few social workers (in the UK) had training in the use of interpreters' (p. 810), highlighting that training is crucial in service provision for ethnic minorities. Serious consequences to ethnic minority children and families can arise if good practice is not followed. Importantly, the extent to which principles of good practice are already in place is likely to depend on the cultural diversity of the area in which a local child protection centre operates:

In [local CSC], because you deal with it so much, it becomes habit using an interpreter [and] explaining what child protection means. You get used to talking the talk. [CW_Anglo]

Best practice model when working with interpreters in child protection

Essential

✓ Children should not be used as interpreters.
✓ Gender-matched interpreters should be offered to observe cultural norms, for sensitive issues (e.g. domestic violence, sexual abuse, etc.) and/or to meet the preference of individuals.

Highly recommended

✓ Translation should be verbatim to increase accuracy.
✓ On a case-by-case basis, offer families a choice between language-matched or ethnic-matched interpreters.
   ○ Language-matched interpreters are better if families fear a breach of confidentiality and 'loss of face' in the community from ethnic-matched interpreters. However, they may not be useful if different dialects make them difficult to understand.
   ○ Ethnically matched interpreters are better for understanding cultural nuances in body language and the way instances of abuse and neglect are described; sensitivity (e.g. for sexual abuse) may be particularly important. They may also be important because of regional conflicts (i.e. having someone from the same culture, not just the same language).
   ○ Some families may not have a preference one way or the other.
✓ Reassure families that interpreters are accredited and that it is mandatory for all interpreters to keep matters confidential, except as required by law.
✓ Provide training to interpreters on child protection issues.
✓ Provide training to caseworkers on working effectively with interpreters.
✓ Respectfully and strongly encourage families to use an interpreter.
   ○ Families may have questionable English comprehension, refuse an interpreter, over-estimate their English proficiency and/or not understand the magnitude of intervention.
   ○ Make clear to such families that even though their English proficiency may be sufficient in day-to-day matters, child protection matters and processes are complex, the concepts and terms used by child protection systems are difficult for any family regardless of their cultural background and child protection systems have the statutory power to remove children (which they may not be aware of).

o   As such, an interpreter is in the child and family's best interest and will assist in more accurately representing the family's voice.

✓   Pre- and de-brief with interpreters so that they are aware of issues that will be discussed and to provide support to interpreters whose own personal experiences may be triggered while interpreting.

Recommended

✓   Acknowledge families may experience loss of privacy.
✓   Acknowledge that families may experience tension between two of their own conflicting needs – the need to feel culturally understood and the need to protect the family's privacy.
✓   Acknowledge that cultural differences between two classes or religions within the same culture can produce biases and judgement in the interpreter.
✓   Strive for good rapport between a caseworker and an interpreter.
✓   Encourage families to bring a support person (that is not a child).
✓   Ensure all parties are heard.

When resources permit...

✓   Face-to-face (rather than telephone) interpreters should be employed.
✓   Allow double time in workload allocation to caseworkers with clients needing an interpreter.
✓   Provide interpreters that speak the languages of all family members.

Unavoidable barriers to good practice that are still good to be aware of...

✓   Booked interpreters may not arrive.
✓   Booked interpreters may have a conflict of interest, knowing the client family, and so are not able to interpret.
✓   There may not be (mobile) telephone coverage in all areas.
✓   Different interpreters will be sent, which is disruptive to relationship-building with long-standing client families.
✓   Meeting interpreters who will not travel long distances may be costly in time and money to both families and caseworkers.

8 To match or not to match?

The pros and cons of ethnic dis/similarity between client families and caseworkers

Compared to ethnic minority client families, caseworkers either have a preference for matching or not – none had no opinion on the matter, suggesting they are (more) aware of the associated pros and cons. Contrarily, there is great diversity among client families: some prefer an ethnically matched caseworker, others prefer a non-match and others still have no preference at all (usually based on a belief that all caseworkers are equally trained, skilled, experienced and/or competent and so their ethnicity was irrelevant):

> *Doesn't matter. Most important, if she's experienced enough to deal with different background, different cultures. [FAM_Lebanese]*

> *They should know what your needs are, they should listen to you. Maybe someone, not even from your background might listen to you, so [caseworkers] all the same. It's a mixed country. [FAM_Lebanese]*

> *[Caseworker]'s doing a good job, so [I] wouldn't change anything. They do what I ask. Everyone is the same in their job, they know what they're doing. Doesn't matter if you're white, black or green. They must get taught at school or whatever, so they all the same. [FAM_Dutch]*

Thus, *choice* for client families is critical to good practice. It cannot be assumed that just because a family is of ethnic minority background they will or will not prefer to have an ethnically matched caseworker.

Case Study 8.1 – Preference for a non-matched caseworker to prove they are not hiding information

Whatever she is or speak, I don't care, because they're doing this job and everyone the same ... She [caseworker] came with Lebanese girl and ask me if I prefer her. I said, 'no, I seen you before, why change? I'm happy with you'. She said, 'maybe you be more comfortable'. I said, 'no, what's here is open to everyone. I don't prefer Lebanese [caseworker] cos I'm not hiding anything'. [FAM_Lebanese]

Advantages of ethnic matching

Overcoming language barriers

One of the most important reasons why client families (especially) and caseworkers would want an ethnic-match is for language purposes – being able to explain themselves fully, facilitate engagement and understand child protection processes:

> *Most definitely the family needs to be given the opportunity to be matched with someone from their cultural background. If they say yes, which they generally will, we need to source that for them. A lot of the time, it's based on the fact that they want to be able to speak their first language to the caseworker. The whole process [is then] more conducive to [their] needs. [CW_NESB]*

> *I can understand you [but my wife] don't have any English, so she can't understand. When she have problems with DoCS, I will come like [an] interpreter. [But] I don't have more knowledge about what DoCS do. So she will ask me, and I'll pass it to you, then you say your word and I'll pass it to her. We keep rotating without getting each other. But if [caseworker is] Sudanese, they can make it direct. They understand [the] ways Sudanese bring up their children, and knows the system in Australia, so she can figure out the right direction you can go in. [FAM_Sudanese]*

Providing cultural sensitivity

Another key advantage to providing a matched caseworker is that they can offer tacit cultural awareness and sensitivity, in turn improving engagement with families and avoiding possible discrimination:

> *If they are the same, there's no need to explain everything of my culture. [FAM_Lebanese]*

> *The pros are the knowledge base, the sensitivity, they know how to approach that family. [CW_Anglo]*

> *That caseworker knows the views, beliefs, of this culture, they've grown up in [it], and it would help. The family respond better, 'oh you understand me'. [CW_NESB]*

> *[Caseworkers] have to understand Vietnamese culture. If they do not [and] just follow Australian culture, they can make the situation worse. [FAM_Vietnamese]*

> *A caseworker from the same culture, going to have more understanding in terms of language and mannerisms, and how they go about everyday life. [CW_NESB]*

I sense there is a difference. English-speaking caseworkers just fulfil what they got to do. Caseworker of Vietnamese origin [has] dedicated more attention to my problems. [FAM_Vietnamese]

Misunderstanding of culture would be the disadvantage. Like, I might think feet-binding is very bad, I might discredit her [mother], [but] in fact she was doing with good intention to provide better care for that child. [CW_NESB]

Case Study 8.2 – Ethnic-matching and cultural sensitivity

I been here 20 years. He [son] was born here. I call Australia home. [But] Australian culture doesn't suit my culture, so I prefer to live in my culture. It doesn't mean I'm against their culture. I respect their culture and I want them to respect mine. We have no problem in 20 years. Except DoCS. Because they know nothing about culture. For instance, most Mediterranean people, especially male, has unfortunately, got bad temper. We got different culture. Sometimes, I am angry, sometimes I raise my voice, but it doesn't mean I'm assaulting you or something... I used to have once a month visit. Many times, no reason, they just cancel our visit. That's why I was angry ... Absolutely [better to have a matched caseworker]. I raised this [a] million times. Because without knowing my culture, they misunderstand me. How many times I told the manager, but it didn't happen ... A Turkish caseworker tried to involve [in] our case but that manager always make sure [to] keep her away from our case ... That woman damaged us deliberately. Somehow she didn't like me, I didn't like her. I'm telling you, it's between that caseworker's lips, your destiny. One individual change your life. Not just my life, my son's life as well. [FAM_Turkish]

Importantly, bias can also come from matched caseworkers *because* of their tacit cultural awareness, or because of regional conflicts:

You have to go case-by-case because [in] some relationships you have to form, that might be the only common ground they have to work with the client, and that can be a very useful way to engage the family. But in other situations, the lack of identification with some of our staff, would avoid bias and opinion and some of that stuff that goes on. [CW_Anglo]

Caseworker to be Sudanese is the main important thing to me. He or she will have knowledge, culturally. Emotionally, you can feel if it is [a] different person. [Otherwise there] may be discrimination ... [But] Northern Sudan is different. We were in a war for 21 years and that's why we are here in

Australia. So if [caseworker] come from Northern Sudan, it'd be worse. Chinese or Lebanese or anyone [is] better! [FAM_Sudanese]

It is also important to note that it is not always possible to offer a matched caseworker:

Ideally, if we had the resources to do that I'd say match [but] it's not really realistic. [CW_NESB]

Definitely better to match, otherwise get the closest mix, [for example] if you had a Cambodian family but don't have a Cambodian caseworker, go for Vietnamese [or] Thai. [CW_NESB]

We don't have the luxury of picking out which case we go out to respond to when there's a level one [but] if we do have a [matched] caseworker, if we have that resource, at least when you are out there, say 'look, we are going to be working with you, what would be best, do you think you would benefit more from someone from your cultural background or are you happy with myself?'. Giving them that option, that opportunity. [CW_NESB]

Pending resources and biases that can occur among matched caseworkers, it may be worth offering ethnic minority families a caseworker of any ethnic minority background because of their tacit knowledge of 'the migrant context'. Having said that, it is important not to stereotype the skills of Anglo and Indigenous caseworkers who have and use cultural knowledge in their work practice:

It is good if we're from the same background and understand each other. We can help them better. I think a lot of CALD caseworkers are more adaptable, understanding of other cultures. They are better at working with other cultures. We're more approachable compared to other races. Anglo caseworkers only know one language. They don't understand that much [about how] to work with CALD communities. They are not that adaptable. [CW_NESB]

Indeed, cultural sensitivity may be less important to a family than simply having a general sensitivity and value for transparency; 'important qualities of professionals include acknowledging they don't always have the answer; not appearing arrogant or superior and being open and honest' (O'Neale, 2000, cited in Chand and Thoburn, 2005, p. 176).

Anyone. Because not all persons the same. Sometimes I have people not my culture who are very kind, very good. Sometimes I have my culture, it's bad! [FAM_Egyptian]

I don't think we should generalise. Every family is different, everybody's personality is different ... Just be transparent with the family, 'look, I know

*you come from a different cultural background. I'll try my best to work with
you and understand your culture. Please tell me if I am doing something that
is an offence to your culture'. Be culturally sensitive and put that out there.
Having that open communication and then being able to do better work. Then
they know you have that level of respect for them – you respect their culture
and where they come from. [CW_NESB]*

It is also important to note that matched caseworkers do not always offer families
the sensitivity they need; they may have extra-stringent interactions or harshness
of manner, for example. As Harris and Hackett (2008) note, 'it is commonly
assumed that a child welfare worker who is the same as the child's ethnic
background will demonstrate less bias towards the client' (p. 203). Korbin (2002)
also says of social workers (in the USA) that, 'even if they do share the same
cultural group, differences in education, SES (socio-economic status), gender, age
or other life experiences may cause substantial communication and interpretation
barriers that must be overcome in a similar manner as if the two were from
different cultures' (p. 639).

Disadvantages of ethnic matching

Fear of a breach of confidentiality among client families

The two main benefits of ethnic-matching are to overcome language barriers and
provide cultural sensitivity. However, these benefits may be offset by the main
disadvantage of ethnic-matching for client families – fear of a breach of
confidentiality, detrimental to the family name and thus an issue fundamental to
collectivist families:

*Definitely not [a matched caseworker]. Not just Ethiopian, not [even] African.
Privacy very important. It's a health issue. I may be suicidal.
[FAM_Ethiopian]*

*Some families will go, 'I don't want anyone from my culture', because they
don't want people finding out about what's going on. There's confidentiality
issues in a lot of ethnic groups. [CW_NESB]*

*Some prefer to have someone who speaks English because it's a very small
community [so] you can meet them at every social event. [If] they have a very
significant face in that community, they feel they have loss of face. [CW_NESB]*

*'Not Tongans – they talk too much, too many problems'. DoCS have
previously sent a Tongan or Islander person to the family and the mother is
reluctant to receive help from them. They would like someone not from the
family culture. DoCS have offered to help a fair bit but mother has not taken
things up as DoCS has an Islander involved. [PAC_case file]*

Thus, families not proficient in English will face a real dilemma between needing to be understood and free to express their needs on the one hand, and wanting to keep family matters private on the other. This dilemma is best addressed on a case-by-case basis that empowers the family to make self-determined decisions (which can change over time and situations). If these choices are not supported, the effects on the client's mental health can be detrimental.

Over-identification by matched caseworkers

Caseworkers are aware of the fear of loss of confidentiality for ethnic minority families, but families are not aware of another significant disadvantage of ethnic-matching for matched caseworkers – possible over-identification leading to minimisation of risk of harm due to their cultural knowledge. 'Identification' allows for good engagement with a family, but 'over-identification' is a risk to children's welfare. It is for this reason that case managers may not be willing to provide a matched caseworker to a client family despite that they offer (overcoming language barriers and) providing cultural sensitivity – a vehicle *towards* greater accuracy in risk of harm assessments. That is, there is a fine line between identification/accurate risk of harm assessments and over-identification/inaccurate risk of harm assessments.

Thus, the reasons why caseworkers prefer not to be matched to a client family are different to the reasons why families prefer not to be matched to a caseworker; different things are at stake – loss of face for families and possibly inaccurate child safety assessments. (Only) caseworkers said:

> *Over-identifying with families is good in a way, to build rapport, but later it becomes a dependency, where the boundaries are very blurred. [CW_NESB]*

> *Caseworker needs to be clear on what their role is, so that the family doesn't identify them as a friend or a support when that caseworker is actually there as an authoritarian figure. [CW_NESB]*

> *Is a person able to put aside their own personal either over-identification or under-identification with their culture to provide a fair and equitable service to the person that they're dealing with? [CW_Anglo]*

> *There is a Pacific Islander caseworker here, who will very much downplay the issues. She will see it as culturally acceptable and we see it as risk. Ultimately, it comes down to the skill of the [case]worker and the manager. [CW_Anglo]*

> *You need [an ethnically] different [caseworker] to have someone who is objective. Definitely consult and go out with [a matched caseworker], but not on an ongoing basis. [Then] the lines between child protection and culturally appropriate behaviour could be blurry. [CW_Anglo]*

> *Sometimes caseworkers over-empathise with their clients, or we might overlook the child protection issues. We'll put our cultural needs above the child protection needs. Some caseworkers want to minimise the issues because they're working with their own community, [and have a] very good relationship with the family after working [with them for] a while. [CW_NESB]*

Thus, cultural sensitivity is crucial for ethnic minorities but the risks associated with over-identification need to be managed to also protect ethnic minority children. Over-identification can cause ethnic minority caseworkers to downplay or overlook child protection matters, which is their first and foremost role and responsibility. However, addressing the issue of over-identification in work practice does not require taking away the client family's right to a choice that best serves their interests. Instead, it calls for good management from case managers. This is because over-identification can occur for any issues relevant to child protection work – caseworkers having being adopted or fostered themselves, caseworkers who have mentally ill mothers, caseworkers growing up in domestic violence, etc. – and in all cultural groups:

> *[Over-identification] happens quite a bit across all cultures, even in Anglo families. Especially cos Anglo families can express themselves a lot clearer and their beliefs and values are clearly known, we tend to be able to relate to them quite well as a Department, [so] we do think about their [parent's] loss, and it can cloud your judgment if you're not really careful. [CW_NESB]*

> *[Over-identification] can happen a lot. Not just with CALD clients, with clients in general in this sort of work. It's hard for caseworkers to distance themselves if they feel a connection or have experienced the same thing, been down that same road. It's part of the job as a manager, to be on top of [it], to be aware, discussing that through supervision. I have supervised Aboriginal caseworkers and they have been pretty upfront and said, 'look I can't go out on this one, I know the family, I know the background, it would be too close to home, I just can't touch it'. I've appreciated that. If they have gone out, they may not be judging the risk as well as what they could have been. [CW_NESB]*

Thus, the sensitivity matched caseworkers can provide, can at any point become 'too blurry' for any group with any issue. It would be the job of a good case manager to intervene, mentor, decide, mediate, re-allocate and/or support both the caseworker and client family with what is best for that subject child (especially when client families transfer their problems onto the ethnically matched caseworker due to their over-identification (Gray, 2003). In short, the preference of the client family is not trumped by the risk to accurate assessments associated with over-identification; the needs of the family still come first, and if over-identification occurs, this needs to be appropriately and adequately managed.

Conflict of interest for matched caseworkers

Another significant drawback of ethnic-matching is that it cannot be provided if the caseworker knows the client family. This would be a conflict of interest:

> *A lot of caseworkers know the families we are dealing with and it might be a conflict of interest. [CW_Anglo]*

> *If you are living in the same area as where you work, and you've grown up in this area and [are] from the same background, caseworkers would find that difficult. [CW_NESB]*

> *There are some really large cultural groups, like Vietnamese or Chinese, where it may not be an issue, [but] an Afghani cultural group, I don't think it [ethnic-matching] would work. Problem in terms of knowing the family. [CW_Anglo]*

> *In an ideal world, matching would be really useful for the clients, but from a casework perspective, if my client is Egyptian and they know I'm Egyptian, there's all sorts of issues about me busting in there and taking their kids. Like that's going to end up at my dad's house. [CW_NESB]*

Korbin (2002) similarly says, 'power differentials inherent in a clinical encounter between provider and recipient may also pose barriers among those that share a cultural tradition' (p. 639). Thus, caseworkers may self-select to not engage in cases of conflict of interest. This is an example of good practice.

Unfortunately, conflict of interest may not always be disclosed by caseworkers and this is an important issue that would need to be managed in the workplace:

> *What doesn't work is when you've got someone from a culture who knows the people but don't disclose they know the people. But obviously they do know [them] because they know where the bathroom is and know how to help themselves to a drink and stuff. [CW_Anglo]*

Not being able to learn about other cultures

One benefit of not matching caseworkers and families is that non-matched caseworkers learn about other cultures. Direct, on-the-job training and learning of other cultures in casework is a critical component of cultural competency (see Chapter 11). As Chand and Thoburn (2005) put it:

> Cultural competency training for all social workers (in the UK) is essential because even if workers are matched for race, the diversity of the UK means that all workers are likely to be providing services to families whose language,

cultural heritage, social background and/or religious affiliation differ in at
least some important respects from their own.

(p. 177)

Not being able to learn about cultures is a problem because if families ask for a
non-matched caseworker – for fear of a breach of confidentiality – then they need
to be working with a caseworker who is aware of and sensitive to culture at some
basic level. They can always consult later for further information, but do need to
bring some fundamental skills in cultural competency to the engagement, and one
way to gain these skills is to directly work with families from a diverse range of
backgrounds.

> *As they [non-CALD caseworkers] become more experienced working with
> CALD communities, they become better at it. If they're new caseworkers and
> don't know much about other cultures, they can become very judgemental
> and make bad decisions. [CW_NESB]*

> *I prefer other caseworkers have the opportunity to work with CALD families
> more. Otherwise we would be just stuck. What if we don't have enough people
> who are from those particular cultures? Then those [non-CALD] caseworkers
> are not going to have the experience or knowledge. Not only do the families
> have to come out of their comfort zone... It's breaking that barrier.
> [CW_NESB]*

The literature also notes that there is an over-reliance on ethnic minority
caseworkers to be 'cultural experts' instead of being informed themselves (Sale,
2006, p. 29). This can lead to tension between ethnic minority caseworkers and
their colleagues. Thus, responsibility for work with ethnic minority families
should not be placed solely on ethnic minority caseworkers; ethnic-matching may
be 'a quick band-aid solution (and) the responsibility for addressing ethnicity and
racism should be shared by all workers, black and white' (Chand, 2000, p. 76):

> *As a manager, it's important to challenge people's assumptions. To say
> 'CALD workers can't interact with Anglo families' is not a fair statement,
> and the same goes with 'Anglo workers can't interact with CALD families'.
> [CW_Anglo]*

Gender-matching

Although not the focus of this chapter, it is still critical to explore whether gender-
matching is in the best interest of ethnic minorities. Sometimes, gender-matching
is not important:

> *Man or girl, that is not the matter. The matter is, if she or he got qualified to
> do that job. [AFR_Sudanese]*

However, at other times, families prefer a gender-matched caseworker:

I prefer a woman because the woman understand more than men, they have more feelings, they mothers, they more sensitive. [FAM_Argentinian]

Has to be man [caseworker]. I did actually ask them, 'please, I need male caseworker', because all my caseworkers female. I believe a man can understand a man. A father can understand a father better, mother can understand mother better ... [But] same culture more important [than gender-matching]. [FAM_Turkish]

Gender-matching may not just be important to meet personal preferences but also to observe religious norms:

We were working with [a] Muslim family from Pakistan, and we did have difficulties engaging the family. [They were] dealing with a system, [where] they were very frightened to express their opinion. [But also] differences in the way they approach male–female relationships. [CW_NESB]

In any culture that follows Islam, it's [gender-matching] very important, because there's certain rules they have to follow. It depends on how strict the family is with the religion [but] generally, a woman isn't allowed to even shake hands or speak to a male that isn't from her family or married to her, so that's very important. [CW_NESB]

Key points

- The two main advantages of ethnic-matching are overcoming language barriers and providing cultural sensitivity. However, not all matched caseworkers offer cultural sensitivity.
- The four main disadvantages of ethnic-matching are:
  - Fear of breached confidentiality among families that would lead to loss of face in the community.
  - Over-identification with families by caseworkers, leading to minimisation of risk of harm in child safety assessments. Caseworkers themselves as well as culturally competent case managers are responsible for managing over-identification when it occurs.
  - Conflict of interest when caseworkers know families and so cannot meet a family's request for a matched caseworker. Matched caseworkers who do not disclose conflict of interest in knowing the client family risk the child's safety.

- o   Not being able to gain direct on-the-job learning about other cultures placing pressure on matched caseworkers. This compromises being able to offer a good service when client families ask for a non-matched caseworker or if there are resource constraints.
- Balancing these advantages and disadvantages best occurs on a case-by-case basis that first asks families for their preference (pending available resources).
- Gender-matching may also need to be considered for personal and/or religious reasons.

Recommendations for practice: Decision-making prompts when considering ethnic-matching for client families

✓   Is language a significant barrier for the client family?
✓   Are families fearful that a matched caseworker will breach confidentiality?
✓   Would the client family prefer an interpreter over a matched caseworker?
✓   Does the local child protection office have the capacity to offer a matched caseworker?
✓   Has the client family been asked if they want a matched caseworker?
✓   Have gender issues been considered (e.g. personal preference, religious norms, etc.)?
✓   Is over-identification occurring (by families or caseworkers)?
✓   Have caseworkers disclosed possible conflicts of interest?
✓   Is the case manager trained in, and considered by caseworkers to be high in, cultural competency?
✓   Have all caseworkers been given the opportunity to work with a range of families to increase their cultural knowledge?
✓   Has a 'multicultural caseworker' been consulted on cultural issues if the family wants a non-matched caseworker?

9 Ethnic minority children in the out-of-home care system

How do they fare compared to Aboriginal and Anglo children?

Reactions to being removed: a universal trauma not to be under-estimated

Children in out-of-home care (OOHC) have been removed from their caregivers because remaining with them is assessed as significantly compromising the child's current safety and putting them in significant risk of future harm. It is understood that the removal of children is intrusive, and is regarded as a last resort consistent with the 'principle of minimal intrusion' (Elliot and Sultman, 1998), unless the harm is severe. Examples of keeping families together and designing long-term support for families were found in the case files:

> *Multicultural CW advised that DoCS could have removed the children this week but we wanted to keep them with their mother. [LEB_case file]*

> *DoCS provided case management to the family around issues of parenting, alternative ways of disciplines and understanding child development for 2 years, and [now] closed the case stating that the issues seemed to have settled within the family. The children are good at home and at school. [LEB_case file]*

> *Caller upset that Department of Housing [DOH] told her that her children would be taken away if she didn't seek accommodation. DOH stated they won't assist mother anymore and will involve DoCS to have the children removed from her. Mother wanted to again confirm that DoCS would not take her children away from her. Advised mother that removal of children was not DoCS' first response when assisting families. [LEB_case file]*

**Example of poor practice 9.1 –
Removing children too quickly and denying restoration plans**

From my experience, if there is injury or harm already caused, we just go straight to removal. We don't look at the whole picture. We are there for one or two hours doing the assessment. We don't really know if this child feels loved in this home. If they have had all the good times, but then there was just that one breaking point ... Some caseworkers have the mentality, 'previous research has shown that children that have been removed [and] gone into the system, when you restore them, it doesn't work, so what's the point? It causes more harm to put them back than having them in care long-term [so] go straight to long-term orders, don't work on a restoration plan. If they get their act together, they can reapply'. Where's the fairness in giving this family a chance? Especially when they are not in a relative-placement, they are in foster care, that damage from one placement to another (it's very rare that they stay in that one placement), that process, is causing harm one way or another to the child, psychologically. The child is damaged by the whole process. We are here about maintaining families. Keeping families together is our focus. We should not be the judge of saying, 'this child would be much better in this non-relative foster placement [because] this carer can put her in private school'. If we can work on this mother, whether she can't provide as much quality of life as somebody else, that's wrong. They've gone through a crisis, they've done something wrong, [but] if they've identified it, acknowledged it, done what they can to fix it, [then] what are they [DoCS] tearing families apart for? That's not what we are here for ... If we can keep them together, in an environment where the child is safe, in [an] adequate [and] loving environment, [then] that's it. That child needs a sense of belonging, a sense of roots. [CW_NESB]

**Example of poor practice 9.2 –
Not clearly defining 'risk of harm' to parents**

I really hate 1998 Child Protection Act, [and how] it says DoCS can involve in family, take the kids, out-of-home care and shit. You know what they say? Simple. One sentence: If they feel [the] 'child [is] at risk'. That's how they took us to court. They said, "child at risk". I said "what do you mean 'child at risk'?", just give me one example. Is there any report? Do you have any proof? In six years, there's no report, then all of a sudden, 'child at risk'. He is a perfectly healthy, intelligent, social, like if I am bad father, he wouldn't end up like that. It sort of speak for itself. I'm telling you, when they got you, they got you. That's why [the] system has to be changed. I talk to lots of parents. It's unbelievable. Like one, they took the kids [when] she was breastfeeding in the hospital. What sort of a human can do that? It's against nature. Something has to be changed in this country. They're acting like a God. Not even third world countries doing that. Australia's democratic and developed country, that's one of the reasons why I chose to live here. But when I actually involved with DoCS, when I get in the system, I find out that it is, unbelievable. If you are outside the system, you thought 'oh everything is perfect, Australia's good country'. No. I agree lots of families out there, junkies, they don't care about kids, I actually agree as an Australian citizen, that there are kids out there who need help. But [the] government have to look at the case individually. Don't put me in the same bag ... You took the kids from the parent, for me, [it's] like they took my arm or leg, [a] part of me. They supposed to help families, not destroy families. I haven't heard one single good word about the DoCS whoever involved with them. [FAM_Turkish]

Families, regardless of their cultural background, report frustration, disappointment, disempowerment and sadness when their children are removed:

NM: Don't take the children away. [CHN_case file]

"I miss my mum, I haven't seen her since court, 2 weeks ago". [CHN_case file]

NF was very focussed on expressing his frustration for the removal of his son, he was very angry. He feels this is unfair. [CHN_case file]

NM does not agree to this addendum. NM is of the opinion that all four children should be restored to her care. NM does not want her children to be separated. [LEB_case file]

Counselling goals: 1. to address the impact of sexual assault, emotional abuse and neglect, and 2. to address the impact of grief and loss from entering care and changing family environments. [ANG_case file]

Caller wants to highlight that child was "very fearful" about revealing this information. Child is worried about being removed from parents, as this happened one year ago through DoCS. Child said this has been the first actual physical abuse by the parents since her restoration. [VIE_case file]

Thus, removal is equally traumatic to the child and family across cultures. The trauma is not greater for ethnic minority children, for example, just because there is a significant emphasis on family cohesion among collectivist groups. While the strength of family cohesion should not be under-estimated as a protective factor for ethnic minorities during a 'strengths and needs assessment', the trauma of removal itself is comparable for any child. This is because the *importance* of family is the same (even if *dependency* may not be):

We have difficulties working with any group because of the nature of our work. People don't like us because we remove children. [CW_NESB]

Case Study 9.1 – The trauma of removal is universal across cultures

Organise a visit ASAP. I'll come see them, write me a letter to tell me when cause I don't want to have phone contact with you, I'll be seeing my solicitor next week to organise to sue use. You have wrongly accused me of being an unfit mother and your sarcastic attitude just will not cut it for me. You'd better warn my mother to stay indoors cause there aint no AVO on her for me <u>yet</u>. I really need to discuss with her as to why she wants nothing to do with me. You have torn apart our family. My kids don't have a mother anymore and neither do I. How would you feel if someone tore your world up, ripped out your heart and trod on it. This is not fair to my children and <u>NO ONE</u> hurts <u>my</u> babies "remember that"! You are a liar, a torment, and I hope carma gets you. You told me I could live with my mum for two months when I signed your temporary care agreement. You said it would be OK. You and [CW2] <u>lied!</u> Liars get hurt. I have a beautiful loving home with everything I need for my children's well-being. How dare you take that from my <u>babies</u>. I waited all my life for my daughter. I thought my life was perfect. Until <u>You lied</u>. I strongly suggest that you take time out to go over all your allegations and see that I am a wonderful mum, and I have never hurt or neglected my babies. <u>Follow Up</u>. To conclude, I am the perfect mum, I never drink alcohol, never take drugs, and I have always cared for and gone to every possible [length] to give my children what they need. Please give me my little Angels back. [ANG_case file]

While the trauma of removal is universal, reactions to it, however, may be influenced by cultural norms, and these should not be misunderstood when attempting to understand family dynamics and what is best for the child:

> *We know so little on how different groups react to grief and loss. Some cultures, they will completely detach themselves, they believe they don't have any more chances. It's then seen as 'they're not interested in child, they don't fight for child, they don't come for contact', not understanding that their understanding of contact is too sad, it's too much for them to take on, to see a child for [only a short while]. [CW_NESB]*

In short, it is important that the power to remove children not be under-estimated or abused by child protection authorities, as parents can experience serious mental ill-health as a result of thinking they have lost their children:

There are lots of different orders – not just removal – that caseworkers can use, like for 12 months, just to scare parents, so that they think twice the next time they go to do something abusive or neglectful. [CW_ANON]

Experiences while in out-of-home care

Abuse in the foster care system

Depending on the situation, removal of children into OOHC can be short or long term. OOHC includes placement with kinship carers – which is ideal, as the child at least remains within its family, community and cultural circles (Barn, 2007; Hackett and Cahn, 2004; Wilhelmus, 1998). However, when this is not possible, children may enter a range of other options such as supported independent living, group homes or foster care. While these options provide safety from immediate risk of harm, there are issues even in these systems:

Neglect by foster carers. [ABR_case file]

Disclosure of physical abuse from foster father. [ABR_case file]

Older sibling has experienced verbal/emotional/physical abuse by foster carer. [PAC_case file]

Child abused by [a] previous foster carer and is therefore extremely cagey about DoCS. [CHN_case file]

Child has an extremely disrupted attachment disorder, having been shuffled from China, Australia and various foster placements, and is consequently behaviourally disordered. [CHN_case file]

Paediatrician: From a clinical point of view, child presents as having experienced disruptive family life with what appears to have been abuse and neglect in OOHC. "I don't like my old carers because they hit me for no reason and I use to spy on them and they smoke drugs. I get very upset when I leave my mum's house. I want to stay longer but I know we are not allowed". [LEB_case file]

When someone tells them [DoCS] something, they've got to take it serious. How many times I rang up saying, 'the kids are in danger, he's [foster carer] bashing the kids'. 'Ok, we'll take that information down'. I said, 'it's not information, it's true, it's happening, I'm seeing it'. 'What can I do?' 'You know what I'm going to do? I'm going to come and take the kids away'. 'If you do that, it's called kidnap'. I said, 'I don't care', and I went and did it. I don't care, I did the right thing. [FAM_Lebanese]

He [son] had eight different foster carers over six years. I just got him back last year. Who is going to bring [back] his childhood over six years in foster care? DoCS made terrible mistake ... The foster parent assaulted my son twice. He ran away, and I went to the DoCS office and had an emergency meeting with the manager, and they said there is nothing they can do. All they can do is change the foster parents. I find [that] very unprofessional, unfair. Not everyone qualified to be a foster parent. They have to be very careful ... My son's last foster parent, I just found out that before she became a foster parent, DoCS took her own kids. How that stupid woman became a foster parent and look after my son? The whole problem is, they dump the kid to the foster parent and don't know what's going on behind closed doors ... 'What do you mean you can't do anything? You are the manager. Fix the problem. That's your responsibility'. They're telling me 'go to the minister'. Which I did actually. [But] nothing has happened ... Kids [are] better off to stay in their own family. DoCS must help that family, rather than get the kids out of the family. It's [the] easy way – take the kids and dump with foster care. They don't really give a shit about what kids actually think, kids' feelings, kids' life. They don't care about family life. This has to be changed immediately. I want a big apology. [FAM_Turkish]

Needs and experiences of ethnic minorities in out-of-home care

The trauma of removal and likelihood of maltreatment in the foster care system is experienced equally by all children, regardless of their cultural background. However, there are some other needs and experiences particular to ethnic minorities that caseworkers should be aware of to best meet their needs and ensure better outcomes for ethnic minority children in OOHC.

The importance of culturally appropriate placements

Child protection caseworkers may acknowledge that culture is important to consider but not necessarily have the luxury of time to do so thoroughly or extensively because of the crisis-nature of the work. In comparison, caseworkers in OOHC (and early intervention) have greater scope for meeting the cultural needs of children because the work is more ongoing:

Our involvement – this is purely child protection – is ultimately about minimising risk. We take whatever measures are necessary. Culture often isn't in the forefront, when it's an immediate-type response. It's the safety of the child. [With] out-of-home care and early intervention, there is that scope to discuss and reflect on it, and work around it in all your dealings. The key part is the on-going part. [CW_Anglo]

Short-term plans in OOHC may also not require significant consideration of culture (having said that, temporary care arrangements can become long term and so attempting to protect the cultural identity of the child should be important, regardless of the initial length of the placement):

> *If it's going to be an 8 to 12 month restoration, then maybe culture's not such a huge issue because contact's going to increase over that restoration. And depending on the age and attachment, and cultural knowledge of that child, it may not be such an issue if they are going straight back. [But] if the child is going to be in parental responsibility of the Minister until 18 and they are only four, then it needs to be the first thing, because that child's going to lose language, community connections. Then caseworkers really need to get it together. [CW_NESB]*

One way to meet these cultural needs is through ethnic-matching. Culturally appropriate placements are in the best interests of the child, and links to a similar language and/or culture should be considered when making placements for ethnic minority children as much as possible:

> *We need to be more aware that when removing CALD children, if we can't find a culturally appropriate placement, then at least try to link them in with something within the cultural community, and not lose that. We do it with Aboriginal clients and we should be doing it with all CALD clients. They are very similar. We need to keep that as a focus. [CW_NESB]*

> *If children put into permanent care [are] not placed with the same culture, which a lot of the time they're not, their cultural identity becomes skewed. They need to hear music from their own culture, all that stuff, otherwise they become completely removed. They have really dark skin but yet only speak English; Anglicised to the point of not being part of their community anymore. Once children hit a certain age they come to these realisations. Things like that make a huge difference, but we don't realise. [CW_NESB]*

Examples of good practice 9.3 – The importance of food

Child at one of the contact visits asked mum to bring Vietnamese food next time. Mum told me she has to bring Vietnamese food every time because child's carer only gives her Australian food and child talks about the Vietnamese food they used to eat together. [VIE_case file]

When you're looking at placement, you are trying to match them up with the same culture. If there's no relatives able to care for the children, you try to find someone who's culturally appropriate. It's good to ask about religion and beliefs, what they eat, what they don't eat. Some people eat halal, stuff

> *like that. Making sure you identify that, and [the] placement with a person who is not a relative or of the same background, that they are aware of that and uphold those beliefs. For example, it wasn't until the kids came and said to their parents 'we had McDonalds and a beef burger' ... I did ask [about] their beliefs, and mentioned [them] to the carer, [but] I think the carer didn't click with Mackas and beef. [CW_NESB]*

Arguably, ethnic minority caseworkers may be more aware of the cultural needs that need to be considered (however, mandatory consultation with a 'multicultural caseworker' would ensure that consideration of culture was systematic for *all* families):

> *I see situations where Anglo caseworkers [in OOHC] are put onto families or communities with extensive cultural needs. I don't think that is appropriate, and I've seen issues arise out of that due to cultural difference. [CW_NESB]*

> *Same [OOHC caseworker] is better, because our culture have different religion, different tradition, different food. Muslim is not to eat ham, pork, drink beer, whiskey. When DoCS take our kids for another culture, our kids, they eat maybe there. We are responsibility for our kids. [FAM_Iraqi]*

There were several examples of culturally appropriate placements (including with kinship carers), or the search for one:

> *In the event that a culturally appropriate placement is not located, the Dept would seek a placement that is supportive of child's culture. [CHN_case file]*

> *Child is currently in a stable, culturally appropriate, foster care placement with her two siblings and one cousin. This placement is providing child with the consistency and stability she requires for all her physical, emotional and psychological needs. It is envisaged that because child is placed with paternal family member she will maintain her identity and also her cultural heritage. [PAC_case file]*

> *PR until 18 years to paternal aunt and uncle. There was some consideration given to placing child for adoption however this plan was not supported by the parents. The placement with her extended family was supported as they were able to demonstrate their willingness and community to maintain child within her extended family. This was coupled with best practice principles exercised by DoCS where child could be cared for in a familial placement where her social and cultural needs as well as ongoing contact with her birth parents could be sustained. [CHN_case file]*

> **Example of good practice 9.4 –**
> **Reporting that culture may not yet have been considered is a**
> **sign of cultural awareness**
>
> *Children initially placed in foster care. No mention made of whether or not*
> *this was culturally appropriate. [PAC_case file]*

However, there may be an unevenness in attempts to find culturally appropriate placements based on whether the child looks visibly different or is half-Anglo:

> *If there's an obvious cultural issue, the courts will ask you to address it. So if*
> *it's an African family, and they are black, the first question a magistrate will*
> *ask is, 'is it a culturally appropriate placement this child is in?' Because you*
> *can see. [But] if that's not the case, then it might fall through the cracks.*
> *[CW_NESB]*

> *When we have a child with two cultures, we give predominancy [to] the Anglo*
> *culture. We say 'that child is an Anglo child', and we place him in a*
> *mainstream placement or we don't put in an effort to find out. We don't do*
> *that with Indigenous cultures. We are a multicultural society, and culture is*
> *more than language and food, it's [also] about behaviour and values.*
> *[CW_NESB]*

The provision of culturally appropriate placements is crucial for ethnic minority children in OOHC for the preservation of their cultural identity and protection of cultural safety. However, a resource issue occurs for ethnic minorities – it is difficult to recruit ethnic minority foster carers because of social stigma:

> *Ideally, placing them within a family that is of the same culture or close to*
> *would be something we would aim to do every time, but it is too difficult, too*
> *hard. [CW_NESB]*

> *We try to provide culturally appropriate service but when you don't have any*
> *Turkish care[rs], and all you've got left on the books is a Filipino that doesn't*
> *speak English, you take the placement. [CW_Anglo]*

> *A lot of the time, cos of lack of placements, you'll find they're from a different*
> *country, different languages, different everything. They try and place as most*
> *appropriate as they can, but they generally just don't have a large number of*
> *[African] people saying, 'yeah, we'd love to care for [African] children'.*
> *[CW_NESB]*

> *We had a Vietnamese or Chinese child, I can't remember, that had a disability*
> *that needed to be removed. In their culture, it's not acceptable for a child to*

have a disability. It means there is something wrong with the family, therefore it's hard to recruit carers to care for, not only children with disabilities, but children that have been removed, because of the whole social stigma attached to that. Being aware of stuff like that is helpful. [CW_Anglo]

I can only speak in terms of the languages and the cultures I know. Some Asian cultures believe that adopted children betray you, they're not loyal to you, [so] why adopt them? A lot of Asian childless couples, would not adopt. A lot of them could become foster carers, but they don't. People also think, 'these children were born from this drug abuse, addictive family. It's likely they will have it in their genes, drug use as well'. [There's] a lot of misconception about what people think about [foster] children. [CW_NESB]

This resistance from ethnic minority communities also complicates being able to provide culturally appropriate placements for children from large families:

Pacific Islander families usually have lots of kids, so how do you find a placement that keeps them all together? [CW_ANON]

If they together that's fine with me, they're not separate. The kids need to see each other all the time. I want them to be together. [FAM_Samoan]

One strategy to overcome the stigma and low recruitment of ethnic minority foster carers could be to conduct educational outreach programs. This would help address the risk that current issues remain into the future:

What needs to improve most [is] recruitment of foster carers. [CW_NESB]

If we put them with foster carers [then we have] to have a right match. Because if we don't tackle [this] – if we leave that for another 50 years, doing the same things as we do now – when I retire in 20 years' time, I [will] say 'things [are] still the same'. [CW_NESB]

However, once they have been recruited, there is great need to support them (Thorpe, 2007). One way to support (potential) foster carers is to be honest and transparent about the difficulty that could be encountered with some children:

It's a difficult job as it is, so people that nominate to be a foster carer, it's a rigorous training process they have to do. These kids are difficult kids. We need to be really upfront with people before we just place them, and not idolise the whole thing and say 'these kids are fantastic children and are going to be great'. [CW_NESB]

It also helps to provide sufficient information about the foster children:

When I first came, they don't inform us much on how to actually take care of a foster child. They never really gave us background information on how the child was brought up beforehand with other foster families, what foods he ate, how he was at bedtime. We eventually had to find out on our own. [FAM_Maori]

It is also important to be aware that some foster carers are less interested in the children than they are in the financial support/incentive they obtain:

I'm a Samoan, I know them very well. All these Samoan, they want [foster] kids only because of money. [FAM_Samoan]

Problem with Muslim foster carers project, the carers only do it for the foster carer's payment, "the bucks", [they] don't care about the children. [CW_ANON]

Foster carers did not meet my son's needs. Whatever he needs, I buy it. Most of the foster parents do that for business. They don't look after the kids for the love. They do that for money. Only little foster parent actually do that for love. [FAM_Turkish]

Additionally, the provision of equal support to foster carers from different cultural groups is important:

Once they come into foster care, they need on-going support because it's a huge legal responsibility [but] Vietnamese foster carers haven't been supported for years. That's a huge issue. [CW_NESB]

The influx of Vietnamese cases and kids that need care is amazing, it's just a huge amount. And we don't have a Vietnamese foster care team but you've got a Muslim foster care team and an Aboriginal foster care team, which is great, it's fantastic, [but] what about these other communities? These issues have been around a long time, and we do complain about them, but these issues are never taken on board and addressed. This has been going on for years ... The Samoan community is huge in this area. We rely a lot on the extended family support network, but it's not always protective. We've required assistance with this group for a long time, dating back 10 years or more. If we're able to meet the needs of other children that are culturally specific, what about these kids? They have that right as well. [CW_NESB]

Most importantly, however, it is critical to ascertain how willing a non-matched carer is to support the cultural identity of their foster child, else there could be attempts to assimilate ethnic minority children:

*There was a case when an [Anglo] carer wanted the child to call her 'mum',
and enforcing a new set of rules, totally disregarding [what] the child was
doing before. Her belief was 'there's no point in you doing that'. She [foster
child] was practising her Vietnamese song. The carer said 'look, you should
be reading. I'll read with you'. In that case, she was instilling within the child
that English was a more superior language than Vietnamese, and it was ok to
forget or not learn or practice the Vietnamese language. [But] that's one of
those few cases. [CW_NESB]*

When non-matched carers *are* supportive of a child's cultural identity (especially
in light of resource issues constraining the provision of culturally appropriate
placements), then the child's attachment to the foster carer is more important than
placing the child with an ethnic-match. If there is attachment, then there is no need
to move the child to an ethnically matched placement. It continues disruption in
their lives and resources are better placed in supporting and educating the carer on
how (important it is) to expose the child to their culture (e.g. food, movies, clubs,
language schools, etc.):

*There is this additional education we've had about Indigenous cultural
issues. A lot of the principles can be applied to other cultures, so we have
learnt in one sense. That has helped, giving us a language to talk about
culture. Good has come of that – good conversations and good questions in
casework in relation to cultural issues. People [are] reflecting and challenging
themselves on the appropriateness of their decisions, about placements in
particular – whether it is appropriate for them to be placed in culturally
appropriate placements or not. [Because] sometimes there is a need for it not
to be [matched] ... Sometimes, there's a third culture for people who don't
quite belong here, don't quite belong there. Where do they fit? There's this
big identity crisis. With good caseworkers, each case is looked at individually,
and sometimes [with] inexperience, people could say, 'they are from that
culture [so] they need to be placed with that culture', without taking into
consideration 'where are the children actually comfortable with?'
[CW_Anglo]*

**Example of poor practice 9.5 –
Valuing cultural needs over the individual child's needs**

*Child is reportedly very happy in this placement [Anglo foster carer] ...
The Dept is proposing a long-term foster care placement that is culturally
appropriate and supportive of child's culture. [CHN_case file]*

Importantly, there is shame associated with the removal of children from ethnic
minority families due to the tarnishing it has on the family name:

They see DoCS as a shameful thing. 'If our child's in another home, what are we going to tell everybody? We're going to have to make up some excuse'. [There is] loss of face, depending on their status in the community. [CW_NESB]

This shame affects contact with children in OOHC as well as the preference for a *non-matched* placement, again highlighting that the needs of the individual child and family matter most:

I don't want my kids staying with these carers because I don't trust them. They making too many stories about me and my girls. They call me and my girls sluts. My kids always complaining about where they're staying. I keep telling my caseworker, I'm not happy about it ... And they want me to go see the kids more, but how can I go to these families where they keep spreading these stories to the Samoan communities? I don't care if they go to Australian [or] other family, but not the Samoan family. Now shame to walk around shopping centres and all that, because when I see people they keep staring at me, because all the schools, Samoan community, they all know about this. To me, I'm very shame about it. I want this to be fixed. [FAM_Samoan]

In summary, it is difficult to recruit ethnic minority foster carers because of social stigma and thus provide a culturally appropriate placement for ethnic minority foster children. In light of this, two key issues need to be assessed: (i) the attachment of the child to the foster carer; and (ii) the willingness of the foster carer to support the child's cultural needs. These are more important to consider than ethnic-matching. However, to also ensure that cultural needs are formally addressed, care plans (short or long term) should be checked with a 'multicultural caseworker' as part of a mandatory consultation.

The importance of detailed and inclusive/consultative care plans

Comprehensive and detailed care plans help ensure that the cultural needs of a child placed in OOHC have been sufficiently and genuinely considered:

Child gets to have a cultural shop about once a fortnight/month depending how often he wants it. Staff are developing a cultural maintenance plan. This will involve looking into Chinese centres and looking for age appropriate activities. Getting DVDs or shows that are Cantonese for child to watch. Celebrating culturally significant days and festivals. [CHN_case file]

It would be interesting to find how much work is tokenistic. No one's actually picking up these care plans and saying 'ok, you've said this [but] what does this actually mean for this child?' It needs to be nutted out on a more practical level in terms of [the] age of the child, links with family, links with extended family, other siblings. Are they in culturally appropriate placements? How much of an attachment do they have to that community? Does that development need to happen within out-of-home care through this Department? It needs to be very clearly addressed [with] really specific questions. [CW_NESB]

Additionally, care plans should be designed in consultation with relevant parties and include their perspectives on what may be best for the child so that efforts to do so are exhausted. Including the family is empowering and tailors care plans to individual family needs (Connolly, 2007; Welbourne, 2002; Thanki, 2007). Also, 'the extended family may play an important role in the rearing of children, but that role is best ascertained by speaking to the client' (Giglio, 1997, p. 6):

We always consult our CALD families because of what's called 'natural justice'. That's what we learn in our legal issues. We have to involve all the family members [that have] been nominated or identified at the interview. [CW_NESB]

When we do a case plan, it caters for the families' needs. When we have a case meeting, you are talking to the family one-on-one, and you are looking at what you need to address. If they are a CALD family, that is going to definitely affect how your case plan goes. [CW_NESB]

You hope that no matter what family you are dealing with, they are involved from the start. They know what you are doing [and] where you are going. It comes back to the caseworker being transparent. It's much easier to work with a family when they know where you are coming from, and you know where they are coming from. [CW_Anglo]

If you can't have someone there to consult with around cultural issues, somewhere fairly early on through your involvement with the family, that needs to occur. Inviting them to participate in case planning shows the family that we are trying to attempt to address the issues in a way that works for them, not in a way that works for us. [CW_Anglo]

However, inclusive and consultative case planning does not always occur. One significant reason may be language barriers:

If it's by law, then we need to include them [families] in our case planning meeting. They are always invited to attend. If required, we use interpreter. [CW_NESB]

DoCS as a whole has got better, in that all families [are] included in case planning. All families are invited to participate but what that means for them, is the biggest difficulty. Language is an issue. [CW_Anglo]

With all the cases that we work on, we try and involve the family regardless. I guess it would be harder [with] a CALD family that didn't have a good understanding of English. Trying to include them in the developing of casework would be more difficult, but I still think you need to. It's going to be a slow process having an interpreter there, but you still have to do that. It's part of our work, we need to engage them. We need them to be involved with us regardless of what action we are taking. [CW_NESB]

Another key barrier to detailed and inclusive care plans, which hinder the full involvement of ethnic minority families in their individually tailored case planning, is time constraints:

If they speak English, it's [case planning] going to be more based on their relationship with the Department and whether they've been engaging. If they don't speak English, then it's going to be based on time and resources. [CW_NESB]

It depends how much time you've got. When we are writing a care plan to go before the court, best practice is to have a care plan meeting which involves the parents [and] all major parties. You sit down and say, 'this is what the Department's recommending, what are your views?' [and] the families' views go into the care plan before the court. That is best practice. [But] a lot of the time the caseworkers will already know the families' views, so if there is not time, they might not do it. I wouldn't be able to tell you exactly how many caseworkers would skip over that, but I daresay that it wouldn't happen every single time in practice if they are busy. If they've got time to do it they generally would. In scenarios where you go to court and they give you a week or a few days for the care plan some stuff would be skipped over. If you've got a few months then generally they would do it. [CW_NESB]

Key points and recommendations for practice

- Because family cohesion is a definitive characteristic of collectivist families, the trauma of being removed could be misinterpreted as worse for them. This is not true. The trauma of removal is equal across cultures. This is because the *importance* of family is the same across cultures. Instead, family cohesion should be seen as a protective factor and appropriately and sufficiently considered when making risk of harm assessments for ethnic minorities. Mandatory consultation with a multicultural caseworker would help ensure the risk of harm assessment was informed and met the criteria of the 'balance of probabilities' – that children *are* better removed than kept with the family.

- Children may be removed from the family for the short or long term. It is particularly important to consider how the cultural needs of the child will be met in long-term placements. Short-term placements can become long term, however, in which case culture is important to consider (e.g. food, music, links with the community, etc.), regardless of the length of the placement. This is true of all children – ethnic minority, Indigenous and Anglo – but particularly for ethnic minorities and Indigenous children because of the systemic threat to their cultural safety.
- Two characteristics of practice in particular help maximise good outcomes for ethnic minority children: (i) culturally appropriate placements; and (ii) detailed and inclusive/consultative care plans.
- The search for a culturally appropriate placement may be constrained or influenced by:
    - whether the child is visibly different (the cultural needs of non-visibly different children may be overlooked);
    - whether the child is mixed race (the combined cultural needs of the child may be overlooked if they are half-Anglo);
    - the availability of ethnic minority foster carers (cultural stigmas make it difficult to recruit a large enough pool). In such instances, offer kinship care in cases of short-term/temporary removal of children, and develop and implement outreach programs to help overturn stigmas in the long term.
- Barriers to good practice within (even culturally appropriate) placements include:
    - Emotional abuse, neglect or other forms of harm (e.g. domestic violence) in the foster carers' home.
    - Lack of honesty with foster carers about possibly challenging behaviour from foster children.
    - Lack of sufficient information to foster carers about the foster child/ren.
    - Unequal support to foster carers from different cultural groups.
    - Number of children that need to be placed together.
    - Foster carers more interested in financial reimbursement than caring for children.
    - Lack of training on the importance of culture to non-matched foster carers.
    - Non-matched caseworkers unsupportive of a child's cultural needs.
- If children are happy in their placement, then attachment needs to be seriously considered. Moving the child from a stable home into an ethnically matched placement is not always better for the child; training the foster carer to meet the child's cultural needs is sufficient and ideal.

- Care plans should be detailed and consult with relevant parties aware of the needs of the child. This approach is empowering, inclusive and tailored to individual needs.
- Language barriers and time constraints may limit the extent to which care plans are inclusive of families' needs (e.g. using interpreters is time intensive and court orders may need to be drawn up in a very short amount of time).

Part III
Wrapping up

10 Summarising the main causes of entry of ethnic minorities into Western child protection systems

What's cultural and what isn't?

Causes of over-representation in the child protection system: what the literature says

Over-representation occurs when the proportion of children from a cultural group in the child protection system is significantly higher than their proportion in the general population (Johnson *et al.*, 2007). It is also known in the literature as 'racial disparity' and 'racial disproportionality' (Hacket and Cahn, 2004). Based on the review of the literature, there are three main reasons why ethnic minorities become over-represented in the child protection system:

1 *Culture* is the cause of maltreatment, which then introduces them into the child protection system.
2 *Poverty*, common among ethnic minorities, increases the likelihood of coming to the attention of child welfare agencies by virtue of coming into contact with other social services (the 'exposure bias'; Chand, 2000).
3 *Biased institutional processes and organisational practices*, predicated on the use of one cultural norm for assessing maltreatment and delivering service ('institutional racism'), introduces ethnic minorities into the child protection system.

Poverty is particularly important because it ensures discussion of class-based, rather than race-based, theories of over-representation (Chand, 2005; Fontes, 2005; Cahn, 2002). 'Viewed through lenses of socioeconomic status, increases in reports may result from the higher visibility of poor families to public and official scrutiny' (Pelczarski and Kemp, 2006, p. 23), and ethnic minorities are disproportionately represented among the poor (Harris and Hackett, 2008).

Socio-economic disadvantage can also impinge on a parent's capacity to parent well: 'whilst there is no correlation between child safety and poverty, it is a significant stress factor, which can contribute to the likelihood of child abuse in families who may have otherwise managed well' (Webb *et al.*, 2002, cited in Babacan, 2006, p. 15). Westby (2007) similarly says, 'economic stress can reduce parent's responsiveness, warmth and supervision while increasing the use of inconsistent disciplinary practices and harsh punishment' (p. 143). Sidebotham and Heron (2006) found statistical evidence to show that the strongest risk of child maltreatment was socio-economic deprivation. Importantly, however, Roberts (1997) argues that 'insufficient, and the lack of provision of holistic, aid to poor families may lead caseworkers to attribute the cause of abuse or neglect to deficiencies in the parent rather than to a passive neglect of the poor' (cited in Cahn, 2002, p. 471).

Class-based theories highlight that (extrinsic) systemic and structural disadvantage deserves attention when trying to understand the needs of ethnic minority groups, without weighting the issue simply towards (intrinsic) culture (Dettlaff *et al.*, 2011; Drake and Jonson-Reid, 2011; Stokes and Schmidt, 2011). However, while poverty may go some way in explaining why ethnic minority children systematically *enter* the child protection system, it does not necessarily equip caseworkers with the know-how for addressing the cultural needs of their ethnic minority clients once they have entered the system. Thus, poverty should not be over-stated as the cause of over-representation or it risks reducing the issue of culture in child protection practice to socio-economic disadvantage and side-stepping the crucial need for culturally appropriate and sensitive service delivery. As Mendes (1999) argues, efforts to eradicate structural inequities in child protection based on class are an example of a macro-approach and run the potential danger of failing to ensure adequate treatment of individual cases. Thus, the notion that institutional racism can introduce ethnic minorities into the child protection system is important for ensuring that assessment and engagement are still culturally appropriate (Hill, 2004).

According to Betts (2002), 'the term multiculturalism has at least two meanings in Australia – tolerance for people of different backgrounds, and active government support for separate ethnic identities and institutions. This second variant, structural multiculturalism, has been unpopular in Australia since at least the late 1980s' (p. 30). Davidson (1997) also notes that 'in Australia, multicultural policies were never extended to include citizenship understood as a bundle of democratic and human rights (resulting in) a silent migrant voice' (p. 14). As Hage (1998) says:

> Each stage of settlement policy has to open up a larger inclusionary space to accommodate a more numerous and a more political migrant population demanding more citizenship rights, more national recognition, more decision making power and more political participation – that is, more integration … In the nature of the dialectic of inclusion and exclusion that forced to open up these new inclusionary spaces for the settling migrants, White politics has tried at the same time to deploy different exclusionary processes to contain them within those spaces … The ambivalence inherent in the White multiculturalism of tolerance and acceptance reflected the way this dialectic of inclusion and exclusion, and its mode of positioning the migrant in the liminal space of the 'not too excluded, but nor too included either', was institutionalised by White multiculturalism.
>
> (p. 21)

Failure to implement structural multiculturalism is an example of institutional racism, predicating access to services and support on conformity to mainstream norms and practices. This in turn can lead to the tendency to 'pathologise other cultures and ignore their strengths' (Chand, 2000, p. 72), as if the issues they perceive or experience are attributable to characteristics of their own culture, and that 'their cultures and lifestyles are inherently problematic and need correcting' (Singh, 1992, cited in Chand, 2000, p. 67). Such biases only further entrench negative stereotypes. Indeed, Chand (2000) notes that 'any assessment should include the likely racism suffered by any one black family and the consequences for them, otherwise ethnic minorities may not only suffer hardship but be blamed for it' (p. 74). According to Barn (2007),

> Social work practice (in the UK) is anchored in a liberal 'cultural pluralist' perspective that precludes a power analysis and a critical discussion of race and racism ... A more sophisticated and nuanced approach is necessary which will involve a paradigm shift from essentialist notions of race that view culture as rigid and inflexible to one in which cultural sensitivity is understood within the context of power relations.
>
> (p. 8)

Gleeson (1995) also points out that the 'ethnocentric design and implementation of the child welfare system is central to its failure to deliver culturally sensitive and relevant child welfare service' (cited in Wilhelmus, 1998, p. 119). In fact, Harris and Hackett (2008) argue that racial inequity in service availability and service delivery is the strongest contributing factor implicated in the racially disproportional numbers in the American child protection system.

Overall, the three reasons why ethnic minority children may be over-represented in the child protection system are not mutually exclusive, and each highlights different but important aspects of culturally appropriate and sensitive service provision. Debates over whether culture, poverty or institutional racism contributes *more* to their over-representation are less useful than developing a holistic approach that can help address the effects of all three causes. As Korbin (2008) says, 'culture should not be confused with structural conditions detrimental to children and families, such as poverty or health disparities' (p. 126), even though 'culture does not work on its own or in a vacuum but in transaction with other variables at other ecological levels' (Korbin, 2002, p. 641).

Cahn (2002) further calls for a re-focus of the child protection system from rescuing children to preventing their abuse or neglect in the first place: 'the debate over whether it is race discrimination or poverty that primarily causes the over-representation of black children in the system, while important, is perhaps less significant than an analysis of what to do about the child abuse and neglect prevention system' (p. 477). Clark (1995) also says:

> The greater proportion of notifications of child abuse and neglect (in the Victorian child protection system in Australia) would be more effectively

addressed by improved social security, accessible health services, more durable family support systems and education and training programs for the children and young people referred – measures to break the cycle of disadvantage.

(p. 23)

Though such a move would not be exclusive to ethnic minority families, they would still benefit from this holistic approach. (See also Chapter 12 on preventive/ outreach and early intervention programs.)

Causes of entry into the child protection system: what this book says

This study does not have a large enough sample to discuss causes of *over-representation*, but it is at least large enough to identify the causes of *entry* into Western child protection systems. Based on the study results (including the literature review), four causes of entry are proposed:

- Cultural;
- Migratory (or 'acculturative');
- Generalist (including poverty);
- Institutional.

Differentiating these helps avoid mistaking non-cultural causes of entry as cultural ones, and accurate attributions have flow-on effects for good engagement with the family. Importantly, the data in Table 10.1 shows that generalist issues are the most common causes of entry – causes they have in common with other families – not cultural ones. In this book, culture for ethnic minorities is seen as synonymous with collectivism and unless the collectivist value for the family and all related values such as harmony, cohesion and honour are directly involved, attributions to culture are inaccurate. In other words, poverty and domestic violence (for example) are not cultural issues, but because ethnicity is so hard to ignore, caseworkers could falsely attribute such things to 'culture'. This is problematic, as it increasingly stigmatises and pathologises culture, feeding the use of false and negative stereotypes.

Having said that, migratory, institutional and generalist causes of entry into the child protection system interact with cultural factors such as cultural norms and values (summarised in Table 10.2), and it is this interplay which causes complexity in child protection work in a multicultural populace. It also means that *all* matters related to ethnic minorities require cultural sensitivity. Thus, it is critical to establish what is and is not cultural in nature when ethnic minority children enter Western child protection systems to ensure accurate attributions regarding child welfare.

Table 10.1 Cultural and non-cultural causes of entry into Western child protection systems

Cultural causes of entry	Non-cultural causes of entry		
Cultural	**Acculturative**	**Generalist**	**Institutional**
Physical discipline (with culturally acceptable, valued or normative disciplinary intent)	Lack of awareness of child protection systems and agencies (especially of their statutory power)	Physical abuse (without culturally acceptable, valued or normative disciplinary intent)	Cultural differences between individualists and collectivists in what 'child-centred' family functioning means
Housing needs (including actual and threat of homelessness, related to cultural factors, e.g. typically large families)	Lack of extended family support or social isolation (so less help available to raise children)	Sexual abuse	Differences between caseworkers in the tendency to remove children compared to educating parents, especially in cases of physical abuse
Differential maltreatment of boys and girls (to protect the family unit/name)	Conflict with parents (due to acculturation)	Emotional abuse	'Parentified' children left with extended family or community incorrectly seen as being neglected (inadequate supervision related to cultural factors)
Religion (i.e. use of religious practices to address family dysfunction, parents citing they are more accountable to their religion than the law, etc.)	Financial issues due to migration stress (e.g. coming to Australia 'for a better life', lack of employment despite having qualifications, etc.)	Neglect (of basic needs, and adequate supervision not related to cultural factors)	
Traditional cultural practices (e.g. coin rubbing)[1]	Fear of deportation or illegal citizenship status (affecting disclosures and seeking help)	Domestic violence	
		Mental health issues in the carer	
		Exposure to trauma	
		Alcohol and other drug issues	
		Financial needs not due to migration stress (poverty, socio-economic disadvantage)	
		Housing needs (including actual and threat of homelessness, not related to cultural factors)	
		Conflict with parents (due to normal development)	
		Gambling in carers	
		Criminal activity in children and/or carers	

Table 10.2 Cultural factors that interact with all four causes of entry into the child protection system

---

Any belief or practice that is seen as culturally normal, acceptable and/or of value

Collectivism
Value for family cohesion and extended family and community
Value for family honour, privacy, saving face and protecting family name
Hierarchical parent–child relationships
Patriarchal relationships
Assigning domestic responsibility to the eldest child and at ages typically younger than their individualist counterparts
Value for scholastic achievement (as a means for enhancing the family name)

Religion (especially Islam and Christianity)

Norms on emotional expressiveness
Apollonian cultures: valuing moderate/modest expression of emotion
Dionysian cultures: valuing relatively more extreme expression of emotion

---

Note

1   Chin (2005) notes that coining and cupping are folk remedies that can lead to misreports of ethnic minority parents as child abusers. A caseworker interviewee also said: '*Every now and again you simply get traditional customs, such as cupping or coin rubbing. [In] one [case], the grandmother [used] coin rubbing simply because he [grandchild] had the flu. Apparently he had burn marks all over his body. The grandfather and grandmother were taken to a Vietnamese GP who advised them that coin rubbing doesn't work.*' [CW_NESB]

11 Getting it right

Personal, organisational and institutional characteristics of cultural competency

What is cultural competency?

The matter of culture and child protection in Western and culturally diverse communities is evidently complex. However, putting the detail into practice requires professional skill, commonly referred to as 'cultural competency'. It is often used interchangeably with 'cultural sensitivity' when intended to indicate an appreciation for the importance of culture in child protection work and for ethnic minorities, and subsumes 'cultural awareness'.

Several seminal definitions of cultural competency are offered in the literature. According to Cross *et al.* (1989), 'cultural competence is defined as a set of congruent behaviours, attitudes and policies that come together in an agency or among professionals and enable that system, agency or those professionals to work effectively in cross-cultural situations' (cited in Brach and Fraser, 2000, p. 182).

McPhatter (1997) proposes a set of fundamental components of culturally competent practice for assessing risk of child abuse and neglect including: (i) knowledge of the history, culture, tradition, customs and value orientation of families; (ii) understanding of social problems, such as poverty, unemployment, truncated education, morbidity, violence and their effect on minority families; (iii) understanding systemic oppression, discrimination, racism, sexism and classism; and (iv) knowledge about culturally appropriate and inappropriate behaviour, child-rearing practices, methods of discipline, nurturing and meeting the physical and psychosocial needs of children.

Korbin (2002) says:

> Although cultural competency is often spoken of as a singular entity, it is many different things. Cultural competency most often refers to practice that is geared towards knowledge of and skills in working with cultural groups other than one's own. It also has a political and activist component in promoting empowerment and inclusion of culturally diverse professionals in decision-making positions. [And] there remains a diversity of options as to whether the provider and receiver of treatment and prevention be of the same cultural group.
>
> (p. 639)

Related to these definitions, Nybell and Gray (2004) say:

> Describing the cultural dynamics of helping encounters without context obscures the extent to which these interactions are structured not only by the worldviews and past experiences of the workers and clients, but also by the beliefs, values and attitudes embedded in and produced by policy frameworks, organisational arrangements and physical settings of social service agencies.
>
> (p. 17)

Thus, across all these definitions, it can be seen that there are three main levels of cultural competency – personal, organisational and institutional (Sawrikar and Katz, 2008). The personal (or practitioner) level includes caseworkers and case managers, the organisational (or service) level refers to the local centre in which the caseworkers and case managers work on a day-to-day basis and the institutional (or policy) level pertains to Head Office.

Importantly, all three levels are seen as necessary and *equally* responsible for the delivery of culturally appropriate child protection services to ethnic minorities. It is often assumed that frontline workers bear the greatest responsibility for delivering cultural competency since they engage with the families. This is understandable because as Chand and Thoburn (2005) say, 'the relationship between family members and the worker, and the personal and professional qualities of the workers, make the major contribution to personal satisfaction for ethnic minority families in the child protection system' (p. 176). While they are 'the face of the system', the effectiveness of their work will be limited by how much support they have structurally; caseworkers high in cultural competency but not supported by their organisation or institution will not be able to reach as many families in a systematic and effective way and improve outcomes for ethnic minorities. Instead, culturally appropriate service will be inefficient and families who benefit from having such a caseworker will simply be 'lucky'. This is unfair to all ethnic minority children and families. Thus, when caseworkers are well supported by their organisation and institution, this has carry-over effects to their clients who will reap the benefits. At the same time, there is little point developing policies if they are not going to be implemented by the practitioners. Thus, a whole-of-systems approach is required; each tier holistically and mutually affects the others. As Chuan and Flynn (2006) argue, the effective development of cultural competency lies beyond the efforts of social workers and agencies, and policies and changes to practice are also necessary for an improved, culturally competent environment.

To aid this, it is critical that each tier be aware of their respective roles and responsibilities. It is also important to note that there is a component of cultural competency that includes non-cultural skills. Implementing these would benefit all families regardless of their cultural background. It also highlights that not all needs of ethnic minorities are cultural in nature.

In short, the most proximate unit to the topic of culture and child protection is the family itself and immediate responses to them when they enter the child protection system. However, the topic of cultural competency moves into a wider, less proximate, layer that surrounds and influences that family.

Personal characteristics

Cultural components

Non-racist practice and attitudes

Perhaps the most important cultural characteristic of cultural competency at the personal level is, quite simply, not being racist. Conscious and unconscious biases of individual caseworkers and case managers that are racist or discriminatory (Johnson *et al.*, 2007), can introduce ethnic minority children into the child protection system at any point during the reporting, substantiation and handling of suspected child abuse (Westby, 2007). It arises from unchallenged and negative stereotypes about ethnic minorities, such as the belief that some groups are more likely to abuse or neglect their children than others or beliefs that 'people don't change', causing caseworkers to have low expectations for the family (Hackett and Cahn, 2004).

False and racist beliefs can enter self-fulfilling prophecies where children from ethnic minority groups become more likely to enter the child protection system and remain there for longer (Cahn, 2002). Maitra (2005) refers to this as 'false positives', where there is an over-estimation of risk of harm to children and incidence of maltreatment among black and minority ethnic (BME) children (in the UK) because of racist stereotypes. Korbin (2008) refers to the tendency to expect and interpret the behaviours of certain groups of people as maltreatment as the 'labelling bias'. While such stereotypes develop in part from 'past experiences, beliefs, assumptions … and multi-generational histories of chronic abuse or neglect' (Hackett and Cahn, 2004, p. 12), it is important for caseworkers to remain vigilant on these cognitive processes, and help overcome the issue outlined by Jackson (1996), that 'the cultural nuances of minority client populations are not fully accepted and are often misunderstood by child welfare administrators and practitioners' (cited in Wilhelmus, 1998, p. 119).

Positively, many family interviewees said 'no' in regards to whether they had experienced racism from DoCS:

> *According to me, they respect our culture. [FAM_Vietnamese]*

> *No [racism]. They've even tried my cooking! Really, it's just open. [FAM_Lebanese]*

> *Yeah, they do understand the cultural background, they do give consideration. [FAM_Jordanian]*

However, evidence of (negative) stereotyping was found:

A lot of caseworkers, not only [Anglo], generalise [and] stereotype people [and] communities; 'all Africans have that needs, all Lebanese have that needs'. In fact, Africans have so many people – Sierra Leone, Kenya, Ethiopia – they've got different cultural practices and cultural beliefs, so we can never generalise their needs. [CW_NESB]

I find [when] supervising [that] there's a lot of assumed and stereotypical knowledge. You have two caseworkers in front of you saying 'this is what I saw in the family' and 'this is what I saw'. It's a struggle. An example is 'a strict Muslim family'. What does 'strict' mean? How do you know they have 'strict' religious views? I find it really challenging when people say those things without backing up with evidence ... So when people are faced with a family that is very different from them, it is easier to assume, 'this is what I know about that family' without really challenging it. It's very easy to do that. It's a very natural thing. [CW_Anglo]

Arguably, age or experience can affect the likelihood of negative stereotyping:

This could be a personal view [but] I think age is a factor in people's views too. I think newer caseworkers come much more open to ideas and learning, whereas, if someone's dealt with a family one way, it's easier to deal with [another] family [of the same ethnic background] the very same way. [CW_Anglo]

While racism from caseworkers to ethnic minority clients is more important in a conversation about cultural competency, since it is what can inaccurately introduce children into the child protection system, it is still important to note that racism can come from clients with ethnic minority caseworkers. It is also important that case managers acknowledge this barrier to good practice, and support their ethnic minority caseworkers:

Anglo families may pick up [on] the accent, and that's the racism; 'what do you know?' ... It's the same with a young caseworker, 'do you have children?' [CW_NESB]

CALD caseworkers felt targeted because of their background. They thought they were not treated as equal as an Anglo caseworker, that clients haven't responded to them because [of] their accent or the way they've communicated with them. [CW_NESB]

I [am] very aware, because of my skin colour [and] I don't speak good English. When I deal with Anglo Australians, I have reservation [that they will say] 'who the hell are you? What rights give me, a new migrant, to remove their children?' I've got qualifications [and] skills [but] I'm waiting for one day [when] someone is going to tell me off. [CW_NESB]

It is also important to note that racism can come from second generation to first generation ethnic minority caseworkers:

> *Second generation NESB caseworkers are little brats. They are little rascals.*
> *Migrants always feel inferior. I see them laugh at the accent of first generation*
> *migrants. After knowing what their parents went through, I can't believe they*
> *do that. [CW_ANON]*

Such occurrences highlight that judgement of others occurs. Social differences in power can create shame and fear of judgement in second generation ethnic minorities, which also plays out as racism. Overall, non-racist practice asks of caseworkers to make families feel safe to be (culturally) different by not judging and accepting (sometimes irreconcilable) differences:

> *[Cultural competency] is not only about showing sensitivity and acting*
> *appropriately, it's also about coming to terms with someone who might not*
> *think like us. [CW_NESB]*

Capacity and willingness for self-reflection

For racism to reduce, caseworkers need to take responsibility for any cognitive biases they may have in the way they process cultural information about their ethnic minority clients. Harris and Hackett (2008) found that 'not all workers were prepared to understand or take into account the impact played by culture or race in their own process of assessing risk or in the family's approach to child safety' (p. 206). They argue 'it is imperative for practitioners to be self-aware and understand their own biases, prejudices and racist thoughts and feelings' (p. 206). Interestingly, they also found that 'professionals who believed the court system to be fair and rational were not vigilant in seeking out checks and balances to racial bias (and conclude they may also be) less likely to seek training or consciousness-raising experiences to address their own bias' (p. 199). As Fontes (2005) notes, 'professionals often think about their client's ethnic cultures but neglect to think about their own' (p. 8). Thus, a value for self-awareness, self-reflection and de-centring the self in the way culture is understood and processed is critical to good practice:

> *A good caseworker means you have that personal reflection and awareness*
> *of where you are coming from yourself; we can challenge our own cultural*
> *biases and understanding. [CW_Anglo]*

> *The majority of us who work here are Anglo, so it's like, 'do we have a*
> *culture?' There's a misunderstanding of what culture means. It's quite a*
> *confusing thing. It's [about] getting an understanding of what culture means*
> *first, before you apply it to others. Anglo people also have culture.*
> *[CW_Anglo]*

You really need to be aware and not let your own values, prejudices and beliefs about other cultures come into play when you are making decisions or assessing situations. A lot of people will find that very hard. There's a stigma associated with each cultural background, but try and overcome that and focus on the job at hand. [CW_NESB]

Example of good practice 11.1 –
Self-reflection critical for cultural competency

When I work with people from Asian backgrounds (Vietnamese, Laos and Thai) I build a rapport very quickly, because I understand their values. I've got more of the eyes of understanding them. [But] I can also be more judgmental, 'how come you bring your children here and you're taking drugs. You're looking for a better life for your kids and now you're like this?' Whereas, if I work with an Anglo family that's got drug issues, I won't ask them, 'why the hell you taking drugs?' I'm less judgmental because I don't have that unspoken relationship that is connected by blood, by skin colour ... [But] because of my work [and] training, I do have that ability to build a relationship with my clients, regardless of skin colour. That [is the] number one thing – come with respect for that person. This job helps remove a lot of preconceived ideas, my judgment. [CW_NESB]

Importantly, self-reflection to avoid racist bias is a challenging and ongoing process with no real attainable end state:

I don't know whether one single person can say, 'I am culturally competent'. If I say that, you have to hit me on the head. There's no way one person who is born in that culture [and] speaks the language, would understand every single thing about traditional values because every single one of us has, inbuilt in us, your own judgmental preconceived ideas. I will never be 'culture-competent'. I will always need training. And it's really up to me. It's not up to the Department to say to me [that I need that training]. [CW_NESB]

Capacity for self-reflection may be constrained by lack of time, rather than lack of willingness:

There are incredibly dedicated, competent, passionate people who are doing their darndest [but] there is no time for reflection [and] good casework requires reflection. [CW_Anglo]

However, overall, self-reflection on pre-judgements that can give rise to racist practice is essential for protecting children. As Harran (2002) puts it, 'it is important to establish the degree to which social care staff are influenced by their own agency value base and belief system during the child protection assessment process ... which may (otherwise) result in the pendulum swinging from cultural relativism to defensive practice' (p. 413).

Cultural awareness/knowledge

Sale (2006) found that 'the main issue ethnic minority families raise is their experience of professionals being unaware of their culture or beliefs' (p. 28). Thus, another component of cultural competency at the personal level is child protection staff having cultural awareness or knowledge:

> *If we could get training to help us have a better understanding of different cultures – regular, identified patterns about things we might face when dealing with another culture – that might be ideal. [CW_NESB]*

Koramoa *et al.* (2002) similarly say:

> While no professional can be expected to know everything about all the cultures they may encounter, efforts should be made to learn something of the predominant ones and how to access reliable information on others. For those involved in child protection such background knowledge is essential if appropriate decisions are to be made. As Lau (1992) points out, an emergency assessment of an ethnic minority family who may or may not be behaving in a deviant manner is not the ideal time to be learning about how members of the culture normally function.
>
> (p. 417)

According to Lee and Greene (2003), there are four 'stances' of cross-cultural learning that caseworkers may have, based on cultural knowledge and cultural sensitivity: (i) *reflexivity*: high cultural knowledge and high cultural sensitivity; (ii) *curiosity*: low cultural knowledge and high cultural sensitivity; (iii) *information*: high cultural knowledge and low cultural sensitivity; or (iv) *ethnocentricism*: low cultural knowledge and low cultural sensitivity. Based on these four stances, caseworkers can make heuristic inferences about the areas in which they may need to improve their cross-cultural practice – sensitivity and/or awareness.

However, the ability to gain in-depth cultural awareness or knowledge is constrained by how emotionally and administratively taxing child protection work is.[1] Assessing risk, managing cases and record keeping are all part of the normal and daily duties of caseworkers, and can constrain their time or ability to make fully informed assessments about the best interests of an ethnic minority child:

> *One of the biggest issues is time. Caseworkers don't have much time to look at cultural issues, because they have to look at other issues. [CW_NESB]*

> *In crisis-driven work you don't always have the time, that luxury of sitting back and saying, 'to what extent is what I'm seeing or saying actually me?'* [CW_Anglo]

> *[There's] not very much [self-reflective practice in child protection] because we are so crisis-driven. It's just bang, bang, bang. You have to make decisions quickly. You don't get the luxury of sitting down and looking at all your cases and go 'this is what I'm going to do now and I think this would benefit'. You are constantly chasing your tail.* [CW_Anglo]

Of those who have worked in child protection programs for any length of time, few would dispute that the work is demanding and highly stressful. Child protection workers must deal with pressures emanating from a variety of sources. They must respond to demands placed on them from the organisation they work for, demands from often hostile and aggressive clients and high caseloads. They are often damned if they remove children from their parents and damned if they don't and further abuse occurs.

(Hodgkin, 2002, p. 193)

Gaining in-depth cultural awareness or knowledge is also constrained by the fact that caseworkers come into contact with families from a wide range of cultural groups, and so it is neither reasonable nor possible to expect them to be aware of all the various and unique needs of each of the groups in the child protection system (Sale, 2006). 'Realistic and feasible demands on human cognitive and emotional abilities' (Munro, 2005, p. 375) are needed:

> *As a manager, I think cultural competency is just being sensitive to the needs of the family and [being] aware of the culture – [just] some idea [of] what our involvement means for that family. If we expect too much from a caseworker we're going to overwhelm them.* [CW_Anglo]

Sense of efficacy to work in culturally diverse communities

As cultural knowledge can be difficult to obtain, it could be argued that having a general sense of efficacy and confidence to address cultural issues, at some fundamental level, is more resource-effective. As Korbin (2008) says, 'the core term "competence" argues for the necessity of moving beyond cultural sensitivity or awareness to developing and promoting a set of skills and knowledge in child abuse and neglect research, practice and policy' (p. 122). It builds, for example, on Starbuck's (1994) idea of competent practice being 'more aptly analysed in terms of the nature of workers' process objectives and their capacity to work within tensions and contradictions than in terms of listings of specific skills and knowledge' (p. 27).

Having said that, efficacy and confidence often emerge from cultural knowledge, so it is hard to disentangle them. As Dewees (2001) says:

The culturally competent 'attitude' cannot substitute for taking the time to find out some very basic aspects (including some acquaintance with the language) of another culture. At the same time, 'learning' some customs cannot substitute for an understanding of the role of culture, of how it shapes (and has shaped) one's judgments, work and perceptions ... It will be far more respectful and efficient to acknowledge the limitations of one's own culture, to ask for instruction, to be led in the cultural ways of our client families. The results will affirm the relationship, inform the worker and validate the family.

(p. 48)

Thus, the terms 'cultural competency', 'cultural awareness' and 'cultural sensitivity' are all related, mutually impact one another and are often used interchangeably despite that they emphasise different things. Together, however, they can promote a general sense of efficacy in working in culturally diverse communities. 'At the very least, the outcome of cultural competency training should foster respectful curiosity about different cultures' (Sale, 2006, p. 421).

Prioritising/valuing culture in child protection work

When practice is non-racist, and caseworkers are willing to self-reflect and have some cultural knowledge and confidence, they will be more likely to prioritise culture in daily work practice. As O'Neale (2000) says, ethnically sensitive services rest on good assessments made by individual caseworkers; 'those who were knowledgeable and tenacious in their consultation with those who are informed about the cultural needs of a group were able to achieve more positive results for their minority ethnic families' (cited in Chand and Thoburn, 2005, p. 171). That is, caring enough to put the tenacity in requires a value for the importance of culture:

> On a practical level, 'cultural competence' means putting the cultural needs of our clients at the forefront of our casework. Identifying their cultural, community and religious needs, sourcing appropriate services, making those links with competent services, educating ourselves on how to work appropriately with people from various backgrounds, having that empathy [and] building rapport. [CW_NESB]

This does not always happen, and caseworkers can disagree on the importance of considering culture in casework:

> If culture is being brought up, some caseworkers get irritated, and then you have another caseworker who's advocating for them. I've seen some of those conflicts. [CW_NESB]

Non-cultural components

Chand and Thoburn (2005) note that characteristics viewed favourably by clients (regardless of cultural background) include accuracy, empathy, warmth and genuineness, and these are demonstrated when the caseworker is reliable, a good listener, honest, gives accurate and full information about services available and agency processes, and puts themselves out to be available at times of stress. They also say that families value a caseworker who is knowledgeable about their specific concerns and appreciate caseworkers who have particular skills, but only in the context of an empathic and reliable relationship. Thus, there are components of cultural competency that reflect non-cultural features.

Empathy and open-mindedness for others

One of the most important aspects of cultural competency that seems to tie all its other features together is empathy for and open-mindedness about (culturally different) others:

> *If you're not able to empathise with your clients, that's going to impact your ability to build rapport and a partnership with that family, which then affects the outcomes for that child. [CW_NESB]*

> *When you are dealing with families and refugees and people that have come from another country, as you go home to your family, you've got your house, your support networks, your rent is paid, you have your food, you have income and you have pleasure in your life. You can't fathom what these people have been through. It's another world. It comes back to that reflection stuff, that ability to empathise. Whether it's Anglo families [who] go through a significant trauma, it might be an inter-generational issue ... Trauma is not a cultural issue. [CW_Anglo]*

The constant and continuous need to be empathic and open-minded can be challenging, but it is nevertheless critical to good practice:

> *People that do social services, that want to help, that are genuinely nice people that care about others, often come from good backgrounds themselves. You don't want to stereotype [but] when you are dealing with the degree of drugs, professional criminals, we've got this clash of two worlds ... That need to be so open-minded and experienced, it's really difficult. [CW_Anglo]*

Respectful engagement, expressed interest, efficient/responsive engagement, regular contact and provision of support and information

Respectful engagement also promotes cultural competency:

I don't expect someone to come here [and] tell the person what he or she have to do. It's nice to behave nice and [just] ask. We are just ordinary people. [FAM_Ghanaian]

Interestingly, one caseworker said:

I've always been out with more experienced caseworkers so at the moment I'm trying to learn what style I'll adapt. Some caseworkers are very police-like in their tone of voice and other caseworkers are more friendly and down to earth, and talk to the family like they are there just as a friend or something, so it varies. In some families you need to be more abrupt because the soft approach will not work. [CW_NESB]

Families also appreciate when caseworkers express genuine interest in them and feel they are getting an efficient or responsive service (including through regular contact and the provision of information):

They take a long time to provide whatever you need. [FAM_Jordanian]

I ask [caseworker for] discount for taxis. Some money this month [will] help. But no answer. Not much interest? Maybe no time? [They] don't do much. [They] just talk. [They have] plenty question for me, but don't do nothing. What DoCS need from me, I do, but they not do for me. [FAM_Serbian]

Sometimes I find things frustrating. When I try and ring my caseworker, she's not always available. I understand I'm not their only case, but I think what they should do [is] have two caseworkers on the one [case]. [If] something arises [and] I need to talk to someone, she's out of the office for four days on a training course, what am I going to do for four days? [FAM_Greek]

Families satisfied with their service said:

They good, because they listen. [FAM_Argentinian]

She [caseworker] always rings when she not busy, and say 'how am I doing?' [FAM_Cambodian]

DoCS work very, very hard to help me. The service is 100% great for me. You have to work with them, to know not to believe what you see on TV. [FAM_Ethiopian]

Everything they do is really good, they take care of us really well, they help us, like calling solicitors and taking us to court, that's good support. [FAM_Lebanese]

Caseworker helps me a lot with my daughter. She comes [to our] home, 'have you done this? Have you tried that?' That caseworker [is] very supportive, very helpful. [FAM_Lebanese]

Having more face-to-face time with families

Inefficient or unresponsive practice is primarily due to the time constraints involved in child protection work that impact on ability to provide more face-to-face contact with families:

> *I'd like more face-to-face contact with families. Take them to the park, the movies. Instead, I'm just at the computer, on phone, it's stupid. [CW_ANON]*

> *That's a resource thing – the amount of time I am spending faxing, photocopying, things like that. [CW_Anglo]*

Organisational characteristics

Cultural components

Having managers that value culture

Beyond caseworkers valuing and prioritising culture in their casework, case managers also need to do this. This helps ensure that caseworkers are structurally and systematically supported in their endeavours:

> *Everything comes down to the manager. [CW_ANON]*

> *Managers have a major role in filtering that [cultural competency] down to the caseworkers. If we are on top of it, then our caseworkers will be on top of it and always aware of it. [CW_NESB]*

> *Depends on which manager is on roster. You have managers who would reluctantly remove children. You have [other] managers who are children-focused, [who] jump in to remove children, we don't have time to look at the parent's history, the parent attitudes to parenting. We don't spend the time to say 'you have a very sad history as refugees or migrants, this is the impact on you in the post-traumatic years, I feel sorry for you'. [Instead] we say, 'you bad parents, because you brought your kids here and you bash your kids'. [CW_NESB]*

Local service centres in which caseworkers and case managers work vary from one another and usually reflect and evolve in response to their local demographic. These variations are critical to good practice, as it means they are flexibly responsive to local needs. However, variation in the extent to which meeting the cultural needs of ethnic minority clients is valued is not in their best interests. That is, some characteristics of service centres need to be the same to ensure equity in service delivery to all families regardless of their locale.

Thus, some community service centres (CSCs) have more open and routine conversations about cultural issues, and such 'organisational cultures' positively affect service delivery and accuracy in assessments for ethnic minority families. When this is not the case, and case managers are not empathic to the importance of culture, there is a direct risk to the child's safety. Moreover, value for culture among case managers depends on *their* cultural competency:

> *I was very surprised that the case manager I had gone out with was freaking out too. I thought, 'I'm allowed to freak out because I'm new, but why are you freaking out?' ... The fact that there's a lack of understanding of CALD families in general [is worrying]. [CW_NESB]*

> *Caseworkers, managers, come with life experience. We've got good and bad. We are parents as well, and [for] a lot of us, our decisions are based on our own bloody private experiences. If you have a manager that thinks that 'hey, this is not my standard, then I'll remove'. [CW_NESB]*

Evidence of how management across CSCs differ in value for culture and its importance was found mainly in relation to the routine use of 'multicultural caseworkers' for consultation:

> *At this CSC, we do consultations with caseworkers who are culturally appropriate pretty well. [CW_Anglo]*

> *There wasn't a focus on multicultural staff here. 'Why aren't we consulting with them? They've got this valuable information, why aren't we using it?' [CW_NESB]*

> *Consultations with multicultural caseworkers doesn't happen a lot here. When I was at [another CSC], it was much easier, much better, much more utilised ... [There were] lots of different nationalities, and different nationalities of workers. It's great. Here, [it's] a different demographic. [CW_Anglo]*

> *We have the multicultural caseworker program [but the] problem is, no one consults them cos it's not pushed from the top. It's not prioritised by management ... How do you stop it from being a token tick the box? Get rid of [the] management and you'd maybe get more genuine commitment to it. I can only speak for this CSC. I've heard [another CSC]'s really good. [CW_NESB]*

> *I wish CSCs use more multicultural caseworkers. They really resent when they are used just for interpreting. They don't say 'what should we do, which direction do you think we should take?', engaging at a much higher level. They feel used. But you also have to change the culture of some managers as*

well. Directions have to come from above. We [are] moulding caseworkers of what they become later. [CW_NESB]

In short, one important characteristic of cultural competency at the organisational level is the equal value for culture across local service centres. This can be achieved through routine consultation with 'multicultural caseworkers', and overcome the issue that case managers themselves differ in cultural competency. To help build capacity in this area, it may be worth having (caseworkers and) case managers doing placements/secondments in other service centres known for having a culturally responsive organisational work culture.

Having enough caseworkers of ethnic minority background and in management positions

Another significant characteristic of cultural competency at the organisational level is striving for a staff work profile that reflects the local demographic (Ahmed, 2004). Of course, 'organisations should not expect cultural competency to emerge simply by having a culturally diverse workforce that is representative of the local population' (Sawrikar and Katz, 2008, p. 11), but it is still an important requirement. This builds local knowledge, with caseworkers being able to learn from one another:

We're dealing with a lot of Middle Eastern clients. We have a lot of Middle Eastern caseworkers here [in this CSC] so we can consult them. [CW_NESB]

However, it is especially important that ethnic minority caseworkers be represented in management positions too, so that they have the power to ensure culture is not at risk of being a systematically neglected issue:

If you look at management, it's all white. People with an accent, who weren't born here, get over-looked. Unless that changes, it's very difficult for the culture in the workplace to change. I don't think it's in all CSCs [but] here, the stuff they do for CALD, it's all tokenistic. [CW_NESB]

Having strong links with community organisations

Several authors call for the need to develop links with local community organisations such as ethnic, religious and/or advocacy groups, or other formal services, to address the needs of ethnic minority groups (Chuan and Flynn, 2006; Sale, 2006; Chand, 2005; Lemon *et al.*, 2005; Walker, 2002). These can be drawn on for advice, support and/or feedback, as well bridging links between families and child protection authorities:

One of the groups from the African community that came to talk to us [said] they would help us link up with the African community but also help the African community understand what we do – that we are not the bad guys and we are just there to help families. [CW_NESB]

Caseworker interviewees expressed mixed feelings about whether current links and relationships with local and culturally appropriate community services and agencies were sufficient and fully utilised. This is an organisational-level barrier that can compromise service delivery for ethnic minorities:

We don't really have strong ties, as much as what we believe we do, or what we should. [CW_NESB]

We've been made aware of them [other local agencies]. But from what I've seen, I don't think we utilise them as much as we should. [CW_NESB]

From what I've seen from our training, they [links] are quite strong. We have training each Thursday and we get different groups come in and are encouraged to liaise with them if we ever need their help. [CW_NESB]

In terms of meeting [CALD groups'] needs, I guess it would be access and linking into external sources, because we're not set up as a translating agency [or] library about cultural stuff, so creating those links with other organisations, like the Vietnamese Women's Association, Migrant Resource Centres and cultural groups, [is important]. [CW_Anglo]

Agencies come in and give us talks on our Thursday morning training sessions. The problem is that we are not actually given the time to develop those relationships. Caseworkers introduce themselves [only] if they think they can possibly get a placement out of this community or whatever the case might be. We establish relationships as we go along, if they are needed. [CW_NESB]

Links to local services can also be hindered by geographical factors:

There's not a lot of multicultural services out this way so we're having to access services from other areas. [CW_Anglo]

Positively, 'inter-agency meetings' were conducted between DoCS and other local community services and agencies, but regularity was constrained by resources such as time. This makes it difficult to nurture good links and partnerships:

We tried to have inter-agency meetings, but the success to get the same person to attend and actually do something, varied, based on crisis, staffing levels, training, court hearings, capacity levels. [CW_Anglo]

> *There are a few caseworkers involved in [the] inter-agency meeting, which involves all the community in this area, criminal activities, child protection issues, housing issues, all the issues affecting the community. Every two months they have a meeting here. [CW_NESB]*

Developing brief information sheets about cultural groups

In addition to links with community organisations, it may be helpful for local organisations to develop brief information sheets about the various cultural groups represented in the locale. Chuan and Flynn (2006) suggest it may be desirable for agencies to prepare: (i) lists of cultural community groups in their area and a calendar of key religious and community celebrations and events; (ii) information about countries, language or religious groups that are tending to be represented; and (iii) information about issues of trauma or loss that might be affecting recent arrivals, especially refugees, who may be represented in the system.

Importantly, however, they should be less focused on cultural information that can 'box' or stereotype families and more focused on information relevant to their current experiences in the Western country:

> *If we had a [brief] community profile on each [culture], that would help so much ... DoCS put one together [on families from Ghana] and I read it cos I had to evaluate it. I thought that was crap because it's not reflective of the families that are here. They're talking about ancient stuff like what happened in Ghana years ago, but not the stuff that's going on with families here – Ghanaians in Australia, how they interact with the community, all that stuff. That needs to be re-evaluated. [CW_NESB]*

Non-cultural components

There are several non-cultural characteristics of good practice at the organisational level that feed into cultural competency at the organisational level. For example, Chand and Thoburn (2005) say that to improve the overall service of a centre, it helps to increase the 'welcoming atmosphere, the ethos of the centre which promotes user participation, the specific services that the centre offer[s] and helpful staff' (p. 173). Other such qualities – namely, having enough (experienced) caseworkers and good managers with stable contracts – were also found in this study.

Having enough (experienced and regular) caseworkers

One significant barrier to good practice with all families regardless of their cultural background is the common resource constraint of staff shortages. If staff shortages were not an issue, staff workloads and stress would be low, and productivity and service delivery high. It would also better facilitate being able to offer a non-matched caseworker if this was requested by an ethnic minority client family. Thus, having enough caseworkers promotes cultural competency for ethnic minority families:

Due to current workload unable to allocate matter for further assessment. [LEB_case file]

Matter has progressed to Allocation meeting on more than one occasion and due to matters of higher priority and staff capacity matter has not been able to be allocated. [CHN_case file]

Whilst not optimal for subject children to witness incidents such as these, further intervention is unable to occur due to higher competing priorities, excessive workloads, and trained staff shortages. Matter closed. [ANG_case file]

In addition to having enough caseworkers, it is also necessary to have enough experienced caseworkers. Families, regardless of their cultural background, seem to prefer not to have young and/or inexperienced caseworkers:

They send a caseworker. She's young, not married, she doesn't know what's going on, she has been a child in the family, not a parent – to care and worry and all this. Older people know … They [DoCS] should work on it. [FAM_Lebanese]

However, as one caseworker said:

Junior staff have to start somewhere. It's a shame they have to learn on real people, there's no practice ground. [CW_ANON]

Pending resources, two caseworkers should be sent so that inexperienced caseworkers can shadow more experienced ones. However, service is further enhanced when they also have regular caseworkers. This facilitates relationship-building with families and also avoids inefficient practice:

When I first started with DoCS, I didn't feel comfortable. But then after, she came back, the same caseworker, and I felt more comfortable. She understood me more. [FAM_Lebanese]

I have seen 15 different case teams in six years. I done the same course four, five times. Each time when case team change, I have to do all these courses – like 'Good Parent' or 'Good Fatherhood', 'Anger Management', you name it – all over again. [FAM_Turkish]

One thing I would suggest is try not to change [early intervention] caseworkers. If it has to happen, ok. It's just really hard, because it's a very personal thing. You're opening your door, your heart, you're letting these people in, and you're telling them so much. [FAM_Greek]

Having good managers with job permanency

Lack of consistent management is another organisational-level barrier to good practice; issues may not progress as well as they could have, had case managers been more permanent in their role. This issue arises due to the high burn-out and staff turnover in child protection work (Healy *et al.*, 2009):

> *We haven't had a permanent manager for a long time. Only my manager was here for five years and now [even] she's left. [CW_NESB]*

> *I've moved around, I don't stay in CP too long. I told my caseworkers, if you are going to last here, take regular holidays and move around. Do a shift in out-of-home care, go to intake, go to another office, you've got to mix it up. You can't stay in the one spot. [CW_NESB]*

> *It's very difficult when you get a different manager. Once I heard they went through four managers in six months. That lack of guidance, it's really hard, very difficult. Not knowing who to confide to – that's a big issue. [CW_NESB]*

Job permanency then affects other good managerial skills such as support, mentoring, leadership and collaboration. Munro (2010) has also noted the importance of managers taking feedback seriously and removing fear to be honest among their caseworkers, and Gibbs (2001) speaks of the need for 'reflective supervision' to address the high attrition rate among child protection workers, all of which occur in a system plagued by lack of confidence in its decisions due to constant criticism of either over- or under-intervening (Mansell *et al.*, 2011):

> *Here, the managers are supportive. They will sit down and listen to our proposals, and work with us to get them approved. That's not the case in a lot of other CSCs. [CW_NESB]*

> *I said to her [case manager], if you have new caseworkers I'm happy to be a mentor. They've got a 'buddy system', but they don't have a mentoring system that says, 'sit down, I'm having this problem, can you help me to do this?' [CW_NESB]*

> *Every team needs a good leader. There's a huge difference between a leader and a manager. Anyone can be a manager, have the authority to boss people around, 'do this, do that'. But when you actually train someone to become a leader, you're actually helping the organisation, you're training them to lead a team. It's a ripple effect. They're [DoCS] lacking good leaders. [CW_NESB]*

> *You hope it was a collaborative approach – if people didn't agree they would be able to voice that and it would be taken on board. [In] some offices, that doesn't happen. Some caseworkers say 'my manager told me to come and*

remove the baby, so I'm here to remove the baby'. That's a huge cop out.[2] *The decision the manager makes is only as good as the information you provide. If they're not asking the right questions and paying attention to the right things, sometimes they get it not correct and we remove children for the wrong reasons and then take them back and we've caused trauma in the process. Some managers say, 'you go out and make that decision, I'm happy to support you', and others wouldn't trust people to go out and make any decisions. If you don't have an open relationship with your manager and go, 'this client really frustrates me blah blah blah', 'ok, you're really frustrated, how does that affect our casework? What does that mean in terms of what service we can provide? How is that going to impact on the child?', if you don't have that, then you're never going to acknowledge your own personal bias or your own personal intuition stuff, that sometimes there's no evidence but you know it's there. How do you get there, if you don't talk about it? [If] you don't have reflective practice, you never get there. [CW_Anglo]*

Institutional characteristics

The development, periodic update and continual monitoring of policies and practices designed to promote ethnic equality are the overarching responsibility of statutory child protection institutions, in terms of implementing cultural competency and providing structural support for both practitioners and client families. However, policies that promote good practice for all families regardless of their cultural background, also feed into cultural competency at the institutional level. Thus, there are again cultural and non-cultural components.

Importantly, when improvements are made, and there are efforts to increase the cultural competency of child protection systems, these should be acknowledged (of course, the need to monitor these efforts is continual and part of good practice):

There's always room for improvement [but] I think we are doing ok. [CW_Anglo]

There's a lot more awareness now than when I started, because of the training, the new processes we've got within this office, the higher awareness, and caseworkers being aware of who our multicultural caseworkers are, as well as a focus from HO [Head Office]. It's heading in the right direction. [CW_NESB]

Right from the get-go, we have it ingrained in us [that] you need to have an awareness of culture. To a degree, we do it really well. We have a high level of cultural awareness. [And] because we are often dealing in chaos, we are much less 'shock-able', [we] learn to look beyond. We've got an incredibly professional and competent bunch of people. When I came here, I was expecting to see racist, discriminatory, narrow-minded, incompetent idiots. I was blown away that it wasn't the case. [CW_Anglo]

Cultural components

Pushing policies that promote ethnic equality from 'the top'

Arguably, the most important characteristic of cultural competency at the institutional level – in addition to developing and widely disseminating policies – is the *continual push* for their translation into practice in the field. There is little purpose in developing policies that are at risk of not being valued, prioritised and routinely used by staff; it is not enough to develop policies – their full availability and uptake is also critical to good practice. It taps into the bigger issue that Hackett and Cahn (2004) point out, that 'unless the institution is willing to change, nothing will change' (p. 17):

> One of the main things that DoCS' multicultural unit [has] been pushing is the ethnic affairs/priorities statements. [But] it's one of those things that – it's great to have a policy in place, but at the same time, the chain of commands is not being followed through. Better communication needs to happen, in terms of feedback, evaluation, checking, making sure it actually happens. [CW_NESB]

Caseworkers primarily noted the lack of routine use of 'multicultural caseworkers' and the need for more training as examples of institutional failure to continually push for the importance of culture (see sections on 'Mandatory consultation with caseworkers' and 'Providing training in cultural competency' for more information):

> There has been training, and it has been good training, but nobody is pushing it beyond that – ongoing implementation of that training, every day. If you've got a client from a CALD background, that needs to be something that needs to be put in your case review, supervision, case plan, care plan, placement. That's an element of everything. [CW_NESB]

> Cultural competency needs to be pushed from the top. With Indigenous families, that is pushed from way up the top. Therefore people are doing things. (Whether or not that's tokenistic is another story.) With CALD issues, it's not pushed from the top and it needs to be. No one's going to do anything down here as long as everyone up there doesn't care about it ... If the managers and the people up the top don't see this as a priority and are not pushing these areas, then it's never going to happen, no matter how much training we do. [CW_NESB]

> The move to the 'multicultural caseworker program' was a massive step for the Department, but now that there's no co-ordinator [of the program], there's no ongoing management or rapport building, no ongoing resources provided, no accountability for people to follow the program goals. It needs

someone that's liaising with the managers and regional directors, saying 'these are the great things that are happening, this is what the multicultural caseworkers have been doing, this is the work they achieved'. There needs to be somebody that's putting that on the agenda all the time. [CW_NESB]

Caseworkers also noted that while several resources had been developed and were available on their intranet, they were also not routinely used or accessed in day-to-day practice. If developed resources are unknown, inaccessible or not used by frontline caseworkers, then this is also a barrier to cultural competency at the institutional level:

People are aware there's a section [on the intranet], 'Multicultural Services', [but] they aren't aware of the content of the material, the information that's available. That's the issue. [CW_NESB]

I know there are a lot of resources on the intranet, you just have to find them. Our intranet is frightening. You can't find your way around it. In one sense, there is enough resources, but unless you can access them... [CW_Anglo]

It's not enough if it's just there [on the intranet], it needs to be utilised, and for that to occur you need to be informed that it's there. Nobody's got the time to [just] look it up. You [need] a training session, 'this is what you can do, this is what you can access on the internet'... [CW_NESB]

Thus, it is critical that the importance of culture be pushed from and by management. Institutional structures set the scene for how organisations and practitioners work, and if the 'structural framework' is not made clear to all levels, there is a risk that the development of anti-racist, anti-discriminatory, multicultural and equal opportunity policies (Barn *et al.*, 1997) will be seen as tokenistic. Ensuring there is an institutional push towards cultural competency is vital to good practice:

Make cultural competency more of a highlight, more than just ticking boxes. [CW_NESB]

Having a specialised 'multicultural' unit

According to Babacan (2006), 'mainstream programs' can fall back on a prototypic model of service delivery because of their large-scale nature, having the aversive effect of homogenising the needs of its diverse client group and fragmenting or marginalising the issue of culture. As she notes, 'it is a well established fact that universal systems cannot treat everyone equally or fairly' (p. 73). Thus, 'multicultural units' are more likely to have the cultural competency required to deliver services in a culturally effective way, provide a point of reference for referral and multicultural resources, act as a source of advocacy for the needs of minority ethnic groups through interaction with the mainstream model and develop social capital by investing in culturally diverse communities, helping to build networks, skills, trust and community infrastructure.

The main disadvantage of multicultural programs, however, is that culture may be seen as a separate issue to core business, implicitly supporting the separation of ethnic minorities from other Australian families. Multicultural units may be criticised as over-emphasising culture, ethnicity and language over other important factors such as class, gender, ability, sexuality and spatial location (Babacan, 2006). Multicultural programs may also be less resourced to deliver high-quality services and/or have less power to influence major change to the mainstream model.

However, choices between mainstream and multicultural models do not need to be made; diversity both within and among cultural groups makes a 'one-size-fits-all' approach not useful. Thus, having a specialised unit dedicated to multicultural issues, alongside mainstream models, can enhance institutional-level cultural competency. It is also important that frontline caseworkers are aware of their respective roles and responsibilities and the resources they provide, else it affects good practice; the two models need to be well-bridged:

We have a multicultural unit, but who knows what they do? I have called them to get advice, but they just refer you to somewhere else. They don't help at all. So you do it yourself, if you care. If you don't: 'I made the phone call, they didn't follow up, too bad'. [CW_Anglo]

We've got the Multicultural Services Unit at Head Office, [but] most people wouldn't use them. Most people wouldn't know how to use them. In the Department, there is a lot of self-education. If you need something, at that point, you'll educate yourself on where to get it, but because CALD issues are not something people tend to think they need, unless of course there's a placement breakdown and nowhere to put the kid or whatever, it's not something that would be a priority on a case load. Obviously, as a 'multicultural caseworker', if they came to me, I could refer them to someone at Head Office, and people would be happy to help them, but most caseworkers probably wouldn't do that unless they absolutely needed to. [CW_NESB]

Developing and providing training in cultural competency

The provision of resources, developed by specialised 'multicultural units', is not sufficient for claiming cultural competency at the institutional level. The provision of regular training is also required. It is a focused activity that gives otherwise busy caseworkers crucial time to self-reflect. As Harran (2002) says, 'social care professionals need a structured opportunity to explore their own values, belief systems and attitudes in order to recognise that professionals and clients are not culturally neutral but a product of their own cultural conditioning and life experiences' (p. 413). Chuan and Flynn (2006) similarly argue that training appears to be responsive to the needs of particular clients or cultural groups as trends in referrals become apparent, but it may be (more) desirable for agencies to provide training which deeply explores cultural identity issues and support strategies in a planned way. 'This is particularly important among professionals who have their own strong faith or cultural beliefs, and should investigate how these influence their social work practice and decision-making' (Sale, 2006, p. 421).

Thus, the provision of cultural competency is essential for providing a structured place where deep cultural self-reflection can occur. The benefits of such training are ultimately for client families. As Gray (2003) found, when 'befriending and participating with (migrant) families, the effect was to overturn stereotypes and defeat stigmas, gaining the trust of families and enabling disclosures' (p. 373). Overall, more training was desired by caseworkers:

We've got information on our intranet about working with CALD and refugee children, but we don't have specific training. [CW_NESB]

Once you do your CDC,[3] that's it, the rest of the training's up to you, and if you're in child protection, fat chance you can get away from your cases to do that. [CW_NESB]

There's the section at CDC training, 'working with CALD families', so there is basic training. In terms of deeper training, I haven't really come across any. [CW_Anglo]

I don't think I've received enough training. We've got one training in our CDC, [but] after that I don't remember doing any other things. I've been working three years with DoCS. Not had one session on CALD issues. [CW_NESB]

If you said to me, are you culturally competent? I would take it as, 'would you be confident and competent in working with families from CALD backgrounds and do you know enough information to go out there, knowing that you'll make decisions based on culture as well as our policy[?]'. I don't think a lot of caseworkers are culturally competent, including myself, and I think it's based on lack of training. [CW_Anglo]

What's really lacking is a push to reflect on your own culture, how your own biases get in the way of delivering equitable service to your clients. There needs to be more focus on, 'what are your prejudices? What's your culture? What do you take for granted? How does that affect your practice?' You have to change the culture of the organisation so that people do that automatically. And you have to be reminded of it, because we all need to be reminded constantly. [CW_NESB]

Importantly, caseworkers receive a lot of training and so it is critical not to overwhelm them either:

> *We get a lot of training in DoCS [but] the problem is, from a caseworker's point of view, we get too much training. Because everyone's so busy, people aren't actively engaging in this training. [CW_NESB]*

Moreover, not all learning can happen in a 'classroom', some of it has to be learned on the job:

> *I don't know if you can ever have enough training around it. [CW_Anglo]*

> *I have to say, at the moment, no [sufficient training in cultural competency]. Then again, you can't really blame the Department for that, because there's just so much we can learn but there's so little time. We should be out there, especially in CP – it's crisis based, so it's really hard to spend all of that time doing training. [These are the] sort of things you learn as you go. [CW_NESB]*

Differences in perception about whether the current amount of training is sufficient are attributable to many factors. For example, it may be that more training is provided to local CSCs with high ethnic minority representation and so caseworkers from other CSCs do not receive as much, or it may be that individual caseworkers want and need more information than others:

> *We are pretty trained up. We are continually being refreshed and made aware of it [culture] in training sessions [by] the Multicultural Unit from Head Office. [CW_NESB]*

> *The Multicultural Unit worked through all these packages last year and re-trained. Now, they're bringing new packages again which is going to target every single region. [CW_NESB]*

It also seems that multicultural caseworkers receive more training than generalist caseworkers:

> *Not enough [training]. [Makes] service providers not efficient because they don't have the full knowledge of the background. If they had training, they wouldn't be needing multicultural caseworkers as much, and they would be making better judgments when removing children. [CW_NESB]*

> *[Training] gives the multicultural caseworker a chance to learn about that [other new culture], but it doesn't give generalist caseworkers [the same]. Really, you need everybody to have access to that. We have all these cases, we don't know anything about the culture, and we're making all these*

assumptions. It's the unknown. It devalues your service. Then you get re-reports and you think 'well something's obviously wrong'. [CW_NESB]

Training also needs to be regular to account for the high staff turnover in child protection work and to be responsive to new and emerging groups in the community:

There should be more refreshers. Once every two years at least. [CW_NESB]

We have a high turn-over rate. The training comes in once a year. If you or the managers are not here during that time... [CW_NESB]

Being a CALD person, I have sensitivity to all cultures. But saying that, there are so many emerging communities that I have very little knowledge of. We need on-going training on emerging communities. [CW_NESB]

[We get] a three hour [CALD] training session. If you did it once every 12 months, you'd pretty much cover every caseworker who came through. It doesn't sound that often, but at least then it's available to new caseworkers. [CW_Anglo]

As training has the main purpose of increasing cultural knowledge in caseworkers, it is best delivered by people from that cultural background:

Having someone from that culture deliver it – because they are the keepers of the knowledge ultimately. People learn from others' experiences. Sharing life stuff would be helpful. [CW_Anglo]

It's important caseworkers understand the issues of their client's background [and] their country's situation, because that tells a lot about the people. If you don't understand that person's experiences, belief system, way of life, it's very difficult. Let somebody from the community come and give us a talk. [CW_NESB]

However, it is also important that the trainer is not just aware of cultural norms but also of the role and responsibilities of child protection authorities:

If we could get someone skilled and experienced with the DoCS system but also with CALD families. [CW_NESB]

I want someone from that culture, [but] not someone that has had a negative experience so that they can say what is wrong with DoCS. All they do is DoCS-bash. What's the point? They need people [that have a] thorough understanding of the need to do the job that we do and provide practical experience for caseworkers [on] how to deal with issues that arise with the families that we deal with. [CW_Anglo]

It is also important that trainers present information in different ways to cater to different learning styles, consistent with the literature that calls for interactive training through role-playing and other ways of practising skill development (Barn *et al.*, 1997; Lemon *et al.*, 2005; Welbourne, 2002):

Our weekly 'practice solutions' training needs to be more interactive. [CW_Anglo]

I'm a visual learner, so I'd rather have someone sit beside me and say, 'this is how you should do it'. Sometimes you need to step away from the literature, and say, 'ok, how can we best put it in practice?' [CW_NESB]

I would prefer a person to come from [an] African culture and give us a talk on cultural issues. [That kind of] training is a good way for us to improve our knowledge of practice, our skills. We can ask them straight away if we have questions, whereas if we read through a document, we can't ask anybody. [CW_NESB]

Interestingly, one caseworker spoke of the need for only general training, perhaps due to the time-pressure associated with child protection work:

[It would be good] if we could have training based on general patterns, how to deal with CALD families, what we need to look out for and be aware of, in general, because it's going to take forever if we say, 'ok, African family, this family, that family'. [CW_NESB]

However, most caseworkers expressed a desire for training on specific ethnic groups, and especially training that was practical in focus so that caseworkers can see how to implement theory:

We should be getting training about emerging communities specific to [our area]. If we were to go to [a suburb] with a high Arabic population, staff should be specifically trained in that, but they're not. [CW_NESB]

I've been to a multicultural conference. It was reinforcement of what I knew already, but in terms of what to apply in case work, I don't think I learned much from that. Everything was more like 'ok, be sensitive when you deal with people in CALD groups'. [CW_NESB]

I think what the Department needs to look at is being more specific around different cultures and what you may face entering a family of that culture. If we walk into an Afghani family, what does that mean? If we walk into a Vietnamese family, what might we face? Be more specific. [CW_Anglo]

There are so many CSCs that deal with one large population of a CALD family. Like, the Cabramatta area is largely Vietnamese. We have a lot of Tongan and Samoan, and then there's Greek at Leichhardt. [We need] specific, more intensive, training based on a 'majority-rules' [in] areas; so we have some idea, so you are not walking in blind. There's no point giving us this three hour training on Italian families when we don't work with Italian families. [CW_Anglo]

I've been around a fair while, so I've had the refreshers and the different types of training. I think it's getting better. The information we are getting is more practical, [and] the resources we are being exposed to is more useful for us. It's not so much just theory-based, we can actually implement that. I think we are becoming more aware and it is evident in our casework – what is appropriate with each culture and who to tap into when we need to make those decisions. [CW_NESB]

At the moment, it's very general training. It needs to be more specific. We get training on working with Aboriginal families, and working with Torres Strait Islander families, [but] we only get 'CALD training' which is huge. That has stemmed from the history of the Department, because Aboriginal [and] Torres Strait Islander families are so over-represented. At the same time, it's not fair to give all this training to Aboriginal and Torres Strait Islander families, when there's Greek, Lebanese, Samoan, Muslim families... [CW_Anglo]

Finally, training should not be focused towards ethnic minority caseworkers. There is a need to increase training to Anglo and Indigenous caseworkers. Indeed, no Indigenous caseworkers took part in this study and this may be because some Indigenous caseworkers think that cultural issues for ethnic minorities are best addressed by ethnic minority caseworkers. While there is merit to this, it does not take away the need for a full workforce trained in cultural competency so that any caseworker can competently work with any family:

You see that people who attend the multicultural conference are from a CALD background. You would like to see more Anglos and Aboriginal people attending because CALD families, it's an everyday issue that we face within work practices. More encouragement needs to be made for people from Anglo and Aboriginal backgrounds to attend the multicultural conferences or meetings. [CW_NESB]

Mandatory data collection on variables related to culture

Another critical feature of cultural competency at the institutional level is mandatory collection of data on variables related to culture, most especially the child's and parents' country of birth and languages spoken at home (Thanki, 2007). From these variables, the child's generational status and ethnic background can be determined as well as a possible need for an interpreter. It is analogous to collecting data on the sex of a child as a way of demonstrating equal value for, and an ability to respond to, the unique needs of all sexes and thus gender equality. It may also be that providing 'better training and guidance to caseworkers who are the most likely to collect initial demographic information entering the care system' (Chuan and Flynn, 2006, p. 21) is required:

> *The only thing that's filled in culturally [at the initial assessment] is about Aboriginality [and] Torres Strait Islander, it says, 'not reported, not stated, not known', in the drop-down box. [CW_Anglo]*

That such data has not routinely been collected in the past in various Western child protection systems was discussed in Chapter 2. Positively, the NSW Department of Family and Community Services (FaCS) made 'ethnicity' a mandatory data variable to collect and input in their database in 2009. Thus, institutional change towards the monitoring of ethnic equality is already in effect and moving in the right direction. However, as a result of poor data collection in the past, where routine note-taking on culture and cultural issues was not part of daily work practice, two phenomena were revealed in the case file reviews: (i) the lack of specificity for how culture is addressed; and (ii) inconsistent coding for the ethnicities of families.

In regards to the first issue: on one FaCS form under 'Have ATSI[4]/CALD protocols been adhered to?' the answer recorded was 'N/A'. Given that the child was from a Chinese background, it is unclear if the reported 'N/A' indicates that the caseworker does not consider the child to be of ethnic minority background (which may be the case if the child was born in Australia, for example, and so it is assumed they are assimilated or integrated), or that they have checked the protocols and based on these have decided that they are not relevant to this particular child. While the intranet contains information and resources that make specific and explicit what these protocols are, these were not referred to in the case files. It may also be that it is difficult to identify exactly what these 'CALD protocols' are in child protection work that is crisis-driven in which there is generally less time for the full and serious consideration of culture, and/or the lack of specificity could reflect a desire to maintain flexibility in casework that can absorb and accommodate culture and its fluid importance as a child protection matter progresses over time. There is, however, a problem if the 'N/A' reflects a decision by the caseworker that cultural factors are unnecessary to consider.

As another example, several case files under 'Cultural issues' reported 'Unknown'. This could indicate that at the time of reporting the cultural issues were unknown, but given its common occurrence across all the ethnic minority case files reviewed, it more likely reflects a systematic lack of knowledge about what *precisely* to record as the cultural needs of ethnic minorities.

Having said this, recording cultural issues as 'Unknown' is better than 'N/A', 'No' or 'Not Indigenous', which were also commonplace in the case files. The last two indicate a failure to understand or meet the unique and specific cultural needs of ethnic minority groups, as it suggests that culture is something that only needs to be considered for Indigenous Australians, as if it is disproportionately more important for them than ethnic minorities. Reporting 'Culture – no' is also inappropriate because culture is not something a person has or does not have, in the way a family does or does not have a mental health issue in the carer or alcohol and other drug issues. All people have culture; it is not a 'yes/no' question or decision:

> *CALD caseworkers need to be taught about Anglo families because there are things that Anglo families say that they miss or misinterpret, like 'I'm going to kill the little shit'. They will freak out, but it's just an Aussie saying. They will want [to] remove for that. [CW_ANON]*

> *Sometimes we go, 'this family is CALD or Indigenous, so I have to pay more attention [to culture] and be more sensitive'. [But] then you go to an Anglo family, and some are like, 'oh, it's just an Anglo family'. 'No, there's a culture there as well'. You have to be sensitive to that. [CW_NESB]*

Again, time constraints and stress associated with child protection work may cause caseworkers to use such 'shorthand' to address cultural issues (maybe even reduce them to language needs as if English proficiency is all that really needs to be considered).

In regards to the second issue: descriptions of ethnicity varied across the case files. For example, a child from the Lebanese case files was described as either 'Lebanese', 'Lebanese Australian', 'Culture: Arabic', 'Culture: Muslim', 'Culture: Middle Eastern' or 'family from a Lebanese background'. The inconsistent coding is not problematic in terms of the descriptions, which are all accurate. They instead reveal that caseworkers vary in their emphasis on race, language, culture, religion, generation or citizenship. Ideally, however, information on all these variables is collected so that information on one is not used to substitute information for the rest:

> *Culture: Islamic and Arabic – all family members speak English very well. [LEB_case file]*

This is especially the case for language, as if it were the only culturally relevant variable of importance. For example, some caseworkers appropriately separated reports of culture and language:

> *Cultural background Lebanese, perfect English. [LEB_case file]*

> *The family are from a Lebanese background and an interpreter is not required. [LEB_case file]*

Others, however, reduced cultural issues to language needs:

> *Cultural issues – no language barriers. [LEB_case file]*

> *The family are of Lebanese descent but do not require an interpreter. [LEB_ case file]*

The same trends of inconsistent coding of ethnicity occurred in the Chinese and Pacific Islander case files, but surprisingly, not in the Vietnamese case files. All were recorded as 'Vietnamese'. No cases said, for example, 'Vietnamese–Australian' or 'child of Vietnamese background'. This indicates that there is consistency in recording of ethnicity for this group, but it also seems to suggest that of the four ethnic minority groups explored in this study, this group may be the most marginalised and future research is required.

Interestingly, the same trend of inconsistent coding of ethnicity was found in the Anglo case files. Reports said, 'Culture: Australian', 'Caucasian', 'Anglo Saxon', 'Culture: Anglo-Australian' and 'Cultural issues: Not Indigenous', each emphasising either race or culture. Of all these, the two problematic ways of categorising the ethnic background of Anglo children are 'Australian' and 'Not Indigenous'. The former has the potential of implying that children of other ethnic backgrounds are not Australian (and this can perpetuate social exclusion, a form of cross-cultural non-parity in service provision), and the latter can imply that Anglo children and families do not experience abuse or neglect because of cultural factors; like in any group, a normative belief or practice of value can underlie maltreatment.

Thus, child protection systems would benefit from a more consistent categorisation of ethnicity, and specifically to avoid reducing cultural issues to language ones or as being only relevant to Indigenous families. If caseworkers are better aware of what might constitute 'cultural issues' for ethnic minority families, these will be reflected in case file notes and there will be less chance of them recording this as 'N/A'. There is a general tendency for case file notes to be descriptive rather than analytical, which may in part be related to the amount of paperwork required of caseworkers. However, notwithstanding this constraint, the success of outcomes is arguably less important than the attempt to at least meet cultural needs and engage with cultural issues in the field, and these efforts should be recorded.

Mandatory consultation with 'multicultural caseworkers'

A 'multicultural caseworker' is more than just a caseworker identified as someone from an ethnic minority background that could be consulted if required. They would have a dedicated consultative role, increasing the likelihood that other caseworkers access them for that purpose, and provide clarity on the roles and responsibilities of ethnic minority caseworkers who have casework but who are not in a dedicated 'advisor role':

> *On the intranet, you can find the list for caseworkers if they are identified to be a specialist in that culture, to consult with, [but] I don't call them to find out if there is anything I need to know about this culture before I go in. [CW_NESB]*

> *There's potential for CALD caseworkers to not be managed properly. There needs to be clarification around 'what is their role in a family? Who do we have to use for consultation? What's the process from here?' I don't think that's communicated very well. [CW_Anglo]*

Above all else, the role of a dedicated 'multicultural caseworker' would be to advise on if, when and how culture is related to the child protection matter and how it should be appropriately addressed to yield child safety outcomes:

> *There'll be scenarios where cultural issues may not come into it, and people that have the skills and knowledge and are providing that information to caseworkers will be able to say, 'this is a generalist issue. Although this family does come from a cultural linguistic background, it's a generalist issue and there is no need to have specific supports in place for this family'. [CW_NESB]*

Maitra (2005) similarly describes the role of 'cultural advisors':

> When attempting to 'unpack' culture in the context of clinical practice (as opposed to academic enterprise) it is necessary to understand how a particular family uses the cultural repertoires they have learned in the past in order to act in the present. This task requires one to temporarily fix the 'culture' so as to explore the literature and consult with cultural advisors and ask questions about how other factors such as social hierarchy, religion, language, etc. influence variations within the dominant beliefs of that culture. It is within this framework that the specific beliefs and practices of the family must be weighed and consideration given as to whether these would be rated 'central', 'marginal', 'idiosyncratic' or 'frankly undesirable' by others within the same group. Hypotheses about function or dysfunction arrived at through this exercise must then be checked through observation and interview, bearing in mind all the time that the family's representation of themselves is likely to be affected by the particular stresses of being under (child protection) investigation, and of policies and organisations that are culturally alien.
>
> (p. 255)

Moreover, a 'multicultural caseworker' addresses the issue that there are so many different cultural groups represented in the child protection systems that caseworkers cannot be expected to be familiar with the cultural norms held by all the different groups they come into contact with:

I guess [cultural competency means] understanding the culture of the people we're working with to a level that we are comfortable with. Like, we can make a decision without having to consult that culture group. I think it's going to be difficult to achieve that. You may be good at some cultures, but you might not have a very good knowledge of others. [CW_NESB]

Even some of us, as professionals and as multicultural caseworkers, get confused about someone from a Vietnamese background being consulted on with an Arabic worker. But it's about the competence of that person, [being able to] provide information [that] gives you some idea of what that culture is about. 'Have a look at this material. These are the bits I think are questionable, but it's some sort of guide'. [CW_NESB]

They would have minimal casework themselves so that they can concentrate on their role as advisor:

For offices that have huge numbers of [CALD] people, you need people in the CSC [whose] designated role is not to carry [out] casework but to provide consultation, education, link you in with services, identify what language people speak, stuff like that. [CW_Anglo]

We've got multicultural workers [but they] still got a full case load. How are they really going to be available to consult? Aboriginal caseworkers have a set amount of time allocated purely for consults. I don't know if that's the same for multicultural workers, so maybe freeing them up. [CW_NESB]

Multicultural caseworkers would act as a 'go-to' person for culturally relevant information on groups common in the local area and culturally appropriate services available in the local community. They would also develop and maintain links with local cultural organisations:

A list of what culturally appropriate services are available in our area would be the most helpful thing, [like] DV services [that] target Tongan and Samoan families, and probably the most simple [to] put together. It would tell you if there's nothing available so you are not searching and there is nothing. You may then have to revert to a generic service, [but] it's better than no service for the family; instead of saying 'yes, I'm looking, I'm looking' and there's nothing to look for. [CW_Anglo]

If knowledge is not used on a regular basis, it's forgotten. So training caseworkers 'just in case' is a bit ridiculous. But having a contact person, designated to a role specifically looking at community development and inter-agency work, finding out what culturally specific services are in the area, and keeping those connections to gain cultural knowledge for caseworkers if they come in contact with those families, building those relationships [like] attend community leaders' meetings [and] church groups, is paramount. [CW_NESB]

Finally, multicultural caseworkers would monitor the extent to which care plans are maintaining culture for children in out-of-home care (OOHC):

I don't hear it's [multicultural caseworker program] being utilised much. I don't hear caseworkers, CALD families gone through the court processes [or] our solicitor or Court Liaison Officer saying, 'when I'm doing the permanency planning or working on the court document, I've called to consult with someone from that cultural background to see whether the contents I've put in there is realistic or culturally appropriate'. If we are trying to be culturally sensitive and appropriate and doing best practice with CALD groups, why aren't we just quickly flagging it with them and making sure? [CW_NESB]

Care plans [for] children going into the PR of the Minister until 18 – their cultural links need to be maintained in a very structured way. That is the most important thing. If that doesn't happen, we are going to start seeing the same problem we have seen in the past with the Stolen Generations in terms of children being taken away from their families and finding out years later, 'hang on a second, I'm Aboriginal'. With CALD families, there's not been that structured assimilation, but a lot of the time that [cultural information] will get lost if caseworkers are not recording that properly. We need a process where CP caseworkers write their care plans. It gets flicked over to someone identified as being culturally competent to check over, as we do with legal. They have a look at it and send it back and say 'change this, put this in, consider this, consider that'. Once that's part of the care plan, out-of-home-care will then look at that and go 'this cultural event's on this day', 'this is the prominent family member', 'this is where contact needs to be followed up', and all those things will follow. That person needs to have that link between what we are doing here [CP] and what they are doing there [OOHC]. They need to have both in the one person. [CW_NESB]

Thus, the role of a multicultural caseworker is critical and would have several key responsibilities focused on cultural issues. However, it is also important that there be enough 'multicultural caseworkers' so that access to them is not hindered:

Having more multicultural workers available [would be good]. I know they are there at different CSCs all around [but] maybe making them more available to [other] units rather than being based at one particular unit. [CW_NESB]

There's only one or two multicultural caseworkers in our CSC [that] you can liaise with [if] they are experienced in that culture. Throughout the Department, there [are] multicultural caseworkers [but] I don't think there are enough of those. Ideally, it would be good to have one from every culture. [CW_NESB]

The biggest thing is access to staff that can provide information around what you might walk into, what is culturally appropriate, like taking off your shoes, which is a silly example, but something like that. We don't have a lot of access to that type of information, and a lot of it is local knowledge, not really formal. [CW_Anglo]

Importantly, mandatory consultation is not always possible in crisis situations, but can still occur later during self-reflection and debriefing:

If it's a case [where] something has to be done right then and there, you don't really have the time to consult. But then you need to keep that in mind after the action has been taken [and] consult and reflect on what you've done. 'Could we have done it differently? Should we be doing something differently?' ... When caseworkers are bogged down in casework, they forget 'hey, maybe we should step back and just consult first'. That's the nature of the work. It's all crisis-driven, it's all very much task-focused. [CW_NESB]

**Examples of good practice 11.2 –
Consulting with 'multicultural caseworkers'**

CW to NM: "Meantime I will talk with a Samoan worker to help child". [PAC_case file]

Multicultural Caseworker Release Request Form: "Phone conference requested. Benefits – advise on engaging with the family". [CHN_case file]

Mandarin CW [that was] consulted advised it is not a cultural practice for parents to hide a divorce and marriage from their children, and described this behaviour as "strange". Child was frequently physically punished for unsatisfactory academic work. Mandarin-speaking CW said that if the father used to be a lawyer he would have had a relatively high status in China and then he lost it when he came here. If this is the case the only thing he could resolve to would be to place expectations on the child. It may be frustration so the child doesn't have the life he has now. Punishment (standing naked reciting dictionary) – Mandarin-speaking CW stated this is not cultural at all – Chinese people do not stand naked in the home. It is not acceptable because culturally, they are more conservative people. She explained it would be an insult, to put the shame on someone and make them work harder. [CHN_case file]

I had [an] Afghani [mother]. I couldn't find anybody [because] there is no Afghani worker [on] our reference list [so] I had to ring Afghani workers from two Migrant Resource Centres to get that information. Apparently it is common in their culture. Some families chose not to do that once they came to Australia, but in their country they put babies in a hammock, tie the baby tight when they are asleep so they won't fall off, and they do that to keep the baby relaxed. They have good intentions. It is just [that] some community nurses were finding it unpleasant for the baby to be wrapped like that. There is cultural issues there. It is normal for them and it is not harmful for the babies. We take their advice on board because they know better. [CW_NESB]

Examples of poor practice 11.3 – Failing to consult with 'multicultural caseworkers'

If it was me, you try your hardest to consult with a culturally appropriate caseworker. Some caseworkers – it comes down to personal views as well as not looking at what's best for the family – [will say] 'this is the service we have. It's convenient, it's here. Take it or leave it'. [CW_Anglo]

In my time here, I have not had a caseworker approach and ask me, 'is this normal that they behave this way?' [It's] just general conversations ... This caseworker had prejudgements of the way the mother reacted and how melodramatic she was, 'she's just faking it, causing drama, fake tears, cry all the time', and me knowing that's just very normal – the way they show their emotion, cry, grieve ... This mum was saying about the [foster] carer, 'my kids don't smell good. I don't think she gives them a bath very regularly. Their skin is dry and they don't put lotions [on]'. She's [caseworker] saying these are unrealistic expectations on caring for your children. I know the Filipino culture. They are really proud of physical appearances and how you smell. They like to put colognes and lotions, especially with little children. She's wondering whether her children will receive that type of care. What's wrong with that? She's lost her children, she's grieving and thinking 'are they getting the same care as what I would do?' So I just said, 'that's very normal, and it's not unrealistic for her to expect that'. [The

> caseworker was] quite dismissive, 'she's always complaining about something'. She was actually saying, 'you are wasting my time, I've got lots of things to do. The carer is doing a good job, I've been doing my home visits, there's no concerns, is there something that you really [need]...?' It's just being sensitive. Something minor, but means a lot. [CW_NESB]

Consultation with Indigenous caseworkers is currently mandatory. Mandatory consultation with multicultural caseworkers for all ethnic minority cases would be a move towards more equitable service delivery. It would mitigate differences in value for culture across local service centres and it would demonstrate the institution's commitment to continually advocate for the cultural (and other) needs of ethnic minorities 'from the top':

> It's [culture] not addressed in a lot of areas. Like when we are sending kinship carers over to foster care training, there's a cultural case planning tool for Indigenous families – and it's mandatory – but there isn't one for CALD families ... We have the multicultural caseworker program [but] it's not compulsory. Aboriginal consultation, you have to do [it], it's compulsory. Which is absolutely fantastic. It should be modelled from that. There's a lot of work that needs to be done of making CALD consultations mandatory. [CW_NESB]

Interestingly, Harran (2002) suggests that to ensure there is no imbalance towards cultural sensitivity as the value base informing professionals' intervention, caseworkers should ask of themselves: 'would the standards of care, parenting and interventions of the child protection agencies be "good enough" for their own children?' (p. 412). Self-reflection certainly has its place, but for a more systematic approach in helping ensure that culture is neither overstated nor overlooked, mandatory consultation with dedicated 'multicultural caseworkers' would be part of good, and equitable, practice. Indeed, operational and theoretical difficulties associated with culture and child protection work only further support the need to make consultation with multicultural caseworkers mandatory so that each ethnic minority family is treated at the individual and informed level.

Moreover, the burden of proof for the removal of ethnic minority children, consistent with the 'balance of probabilities' that the NSW Children's court asks of caseworkers, can only really be met if consultation with a 'multicultural caseworker' has occurred. That is, if caseworkers have not made assessments in consultation with multicultural caseworkers (especially if they are not sufficiently trained and have knowledge on cultural issues themselves), they are then deemed as not having met their burden of proof to justify their assessment and decision. And an *informed* 'balance of probabilities' should be a part of good practice for all children, regardless of their cultural background, to protect their best interests.

Development and provision of outreach/preventative programs

Clark (1995) long ago pointed out of the child protection system in the state of Victoria in Australia:

> Between 1993–4, 600 caseworkers sifted through 26,622 notifications, for whom only 6,024 were substantiated as situations of risk. But the 20,000 children who did not warrant full protective action and who only received a limited response are still disadvantaged and deprived and have limited life chances ... With its emphasis on time limited investigation and court action where necessary, the Child Protection Service is geared to short term intervention, as if anticipating a revolution of the family's situation within a matter of months. This can only be regarded as wishful thinking ... Many families will experience chronic multiple crises over a long period of time.
>
> (p. 22)

These trends remain in spite of the more recent development of preventative services because mandatory reporting makes the statistics difficult to interpret. For example, Bromfield and Holzer (2008) report that per 1,000 children, the rate of total notifications in the NSW child protection system between 2000–01 and 2006–07 exhibited an overall increase of 364 per cent, the rate of total investigations exhibited an overall increase of 352 per cent and the rate of total substantiations exhibited an overall increase of 394 per cent. These all indicate high and increased demand on child protection services. However, they do not negate the effect of preventative programs.

The shift towards resourcing early intervention, as a way of meeting the needs of children and families that fall below thresholds of risk but still need longer-term support, has been steadily growing in Western countries for some time (Tomison, 2001; Hawkins and Briggs, 1999). Of course, the paradigm shift from reactive to preventative will take time to evolve and develop, but 'refocusing the system on supporting families and not on failing individual parents' (Roberts, 1997, cited in Cahn, 2002, p. 473), is a worthy end goal. When child protection systems provide early intervention programs, they can 'result in the prevention of local authority care, reduce the need for child protection case conferences or care proceedings, help empower family members and thus contribute to increased self efficacy, improve outcomes for children and their families and improve relationships between statutory agencies and families' (Chand and Thoburn, 2005, p. 175).

Thus, another feature of cultural competency at the institutional level is the provision of outreach/preventative programs. Brighter Futures (BF) is one such program. It is a voluntary and early intervention program designed by FaCS, introduced in 2006, which targets families at risk of entering the child protection system with service provision (e.g. home visiting, child care, etc.) and support in developing education in positive parenting and insight into poor parenting behaviours.

While early intervention programs intended to prevent entry into the child protection system can help all families, regardless of their cultural background, outreach programs specific to ethnic minorities may also need to be developed and implemented at a more large-scale, systematic and strategic level (Reisig and Miller, 2009). Specifically they would need to address the issue that there is generally low awareness of child protection authorities:

> *[CALD] families should be told about DoCS' laws, because most of them don't trust authority. [CW_NESB]*

> *They don't understand why we are knocking on their door. It's important to get out there and make it known. [CW_NESB]*

These information-raising campaigns need to be interactive and delivered while families are not under stress to be most effective:

> *[CALD families] need interactive education, rather than [just] getting information. They don't read the pamphlets we give them. [CW_NESB]*

> *Depending on the urgency, parents are in such a highly strung state that they're not understanding anything new. It [preventative education] needs to be done at a time when they're calm, when they've got time to give you, [and] they're open to it. [CW_NESB]*

> *Having BBQs at schools is creative, interactive, since they're [parents] all there. Parents will obviously liaise with their relatives and their family friends. They start talking, 'oh no, you've got a misconception about DoCS. This is what we were told'. [CW_NESB]*

Deliberately targeting ethnic minority communities, to increase their awareness of child protection matters and systems (Giglio, 1997), using culturally sensitive staff (Westby, 2007; Gilligan and Akhtar, 2006), can help their increased awareness and utilisation of services and programs, break down barriers to access such as language, culture, trust and/or fear (Babacan, 2006), and offset their possible later over-representation:

> *Yes, that's useful to us [community education/out-reach about DoCS]. If we leave children for [a] few years, the crime will raise, and if we have something to resolve this, the crime will reduce and it will give us peaceful life, parents and the kids. [FAM_Sudanese]*

Some preventative measures are already in place for refugees:

> *When refugees and migrants come, they have a quick spiel about child protection laws and the system here, like 'not allowed to hit your children,*

otherwise this will be reported to the authorities, and this is against the law'. [But] I don't know the level or depth of the knowledge they are handing down. [CW_NESB]

It should be acknowledged, however, that the effectiveness of outreach programs may be capped by a lack of real understanding until a family is involved with the system:

When these people arrive, there's all this information. You can't digest it until you really get involved with DoCS. That's when you learn. [CW_NESB]

A lot of our clients will alter their responses to meet criteria they know DoCS would accept, but CALD communities don't have that knowledge to be able to do that. So in years to come I wouldn't be surprised [if] a lot of these new emerging communities are overrepresented for reasons like that. They've got no concept of the appropriateness of their responses and of our role, and as much as we explain that to them, it's [just] not familiar. [CW_NESB]

Nevertheless, outreach programs are essential for helping to address families' lack of awareness, fear and/or misconception of child protection authorities and ensuing possible over-representation later. Funding such preventative approaches is essential to child welfare:

We don't wanna spend the dollars [so] it's a full circle. Put it up here first rather than back here in care – prevention and education. [CW_NESB]

Non-cultural components

Not having an open-plan office structure

Open-plan office structures may not be conducive to good practice. Head Office would be responsible for ensuring all local service centres are designed in a uniform way:

It's abominable [an open plan office]. I can't [work like this]. Often, if you are a person who is sensitive to noise you need to work late at night when people are gone, or come in early in the morning, because you just can't function with the level of reports we need to write and assessments that we need to do, in an open plan environment. It's atrocious. [CW_Anglo]

Perceived equity in workload between local service centres and Head Office

Uneven workloads perceived by frontline caseworkers can lead to workplace issues that compromise the efficiency and effectiveness of the whole system. The ripple effect unfortunately is on client families. Thus, this barrier to good practice also needs to be addressed to improve cultural competency at the institutional level:

> *Only the caseworkers and the Client Intake Manager know the real issues. The people at Head Office have no idea. [CW_ANON]*

> *It's a really sensitive point – the amount of work we do is ridiculous. You see people [from] Head Office walking out the door at 5 o'clock ... [It's a] frustration for me, particularly in CP, [to see] what an un-level playing field it is ... Everyone knows CP is the frontline [and] new policies continue to be brought in for CP workers to implement [but] it's like you are flogging a dead horse. Until they can review the business process of what this role entails, the system is going to be broken and you need to fix that first. [CW_Anglo]*

Positive images of child protection authorities in the media

Finally, improving engagement with families, regardless of their cultural background, requires positive media coverage of child protection workers and authorities:

> *They [families] should have another mentality about us [DoCS] – that we can help them, not just taking their kids. [CW_NESB]*

> *There's no good news stories [in the media] of 'this is what we can do, how we can help'. It's all negative. [CW_NESB]*

> *[When] DoCS come to your home you don't exactly go, 'hi, come in for a cup of tea'. The whole negative image we have affects every family we deal with. [CW_NESB]*

Key points and recommendations for practice

- 'Cultural competency':
  - is an ongoing skill, with no end state, on working effectively in culturally diverse communities.
  - develops from cultural knowledge (or awareness) of different groups, obtained through training and on-the-job learning.
  - is comprised of three equally responsible levels – personal/ practitioner, organisational/service and institutional/policy – critical for efficient and effective practice with ethnic minorities.

- Cultural competency at the personal level requires:
  - cultural components of good practice, including:
    - non-racist practice and attitudes;
    - capacity/willingness for self-reflection;
    - having cultural awareness/knowledge;
    - having a sense of efficacy to work in culturally diverse communities;
    - prioritising/valuing culture in child protection work;
  - non-cultural components of good practice, including:
    - having empathy and open-mindedness for others;
    - respectful engagement, expressed interest, efficient/responsive practice, regular contact and the provision of support and information;
    - having face-to-face time to engage with families.
- Cultural competency at the organisational level requires:
  - cultural components of good practice, including:
    - managers that value culture;
    - strong links with community organisations;
    - having enough ethnic minority caseworkers, especially in management positions;
  - non-cultural components of good practice, including:
    - having enough experienced and regular caseworkers;
    - managers with job permanency and good leadership, mentoring, supportive and collaborative skills.
- Cultural competency at the institutional level requires:
  - cultural components of good practice, including:
    - continual push of policies and practice resources that promote ethnic equality, cultural competency and the importance of culture from 'the top';
    - developing and providing regular training in cultural competency;
    - mandatory data collection on all variables related to culture;
    - mandatory consultation with 'multicultural caseworkers';
    - development and provision of outreach/preventative programs;
  - non-cultural components of good practice, including:
    - not having an open-plan office structure;
    - equity in workload between frontline caseworkers and workers at Head Office;
    - positive images of child protection authorities in the media.

Notes

1 Evans, S., Huxley, P., Gately, C., Webber, M., Mears, A., Pajak, S., Medina, J., Kendall, T. and Katona, C. (2006). Mental health, burnout and job satisfaction among mental health social workers in England and Wales. *The British Journal of Psychiatry, 188(1)*, 75–80.
2 Whittaker (2011) also notes that upward delegation – 'I'll have to talk to my manager about that' – is a social defence within organisations made by individual caseworkers to reduce anxiety provoked by the need to make decisions.
3 Caseworker Development Course.
4 Aboriginal and Torres Strait Islander (ATSI).

12 Conclusion and where to from here?

Equality and equity: bringing it all together into 'a final word'

The most fundamental theoretical debate in all cross-cultural research is that between 'emic' and 'etic' approaches to data analysis. The debate represents opposite ends of a methodological dilemma for researchers and underpins the validity of findings.

The emic approach is relativist, aligns with social constructionism and represents the view that culture is unique to a group and qualitative in nature so different groups cannot and should not be compared. It values the way groups speak about and make sense of themselves (and thus autonomy and self-determination), and thus belies that all groups are equal. It avoids using characteristics of one group to make sense of another group and false judgements that a group is 'lacking' on something that may not even be relevant to them.

The etic approach is absolutist, aligns with objective empiricism and represents the view that while groups may be different in their values, norms and beliefs, they still have access to the same, universal rights and opportunities. To be able to identify which groups have poorer access to these rights and opportunities, cross-cultural comparisons that place all groups on the same set of axes need to be made.

Each approach offers what the other cannot because they have two different end goals: above all else, the emic approach values equality and the etic approach values equity. Both are in fact necessary. To that end, two conclusive points are made regarding the promotion of child safety for children from ethnic minority groups:

1 Ethnic minorities need to be understood within a 'lens' that is relevant to them (and only them), as this promotes equality.
2 Ethnic minorities need to receive the same service elements that protect cultural safety that Indigenous groups currently receive, as this promotes equity.

Together, these will ensure that some non-definable combination of 'absolutism' and 'relativism', on a case-by-case basis, is used to assess ethnic minority children by child protection workers fully aware and appreciative of the risks of both ends of the continuum. They ensure that the importance of culture is not overlooked, downplayed, under-estimated or over-stated during any assessment and decision-making stages:

> *'Ideal model'? That's where it's flawed, there's no ideal model. In reality, 'theory-practice structure' doesn't come in a neat tidy box, it's not black or white (sic), so whatever model you have is going to have to be flexible and adaptable to the ongoing, changing needs of the case as it develops. [CW_Anglo]*

Equality: using the right 'lens'

In the same way that Indigenous people have a unique story that shapes and frames their context in a Western child protection system, so too do ethnic minorities. The right 'lens' must be used to make appropriate sense of their needs and experiences in the child protection system. In other words, each group has their own 'story' and if caseworkers are not aware of or sensitive to it, then they will not be able to deliver best practice. If a caseworker was not aware of the 'Stolen Generations', for example, their ability to help an individual Indigenous family would be grossly compromised.

The unique 'story' for ethnic minorities is that some of their harmful parenting behaviours are determined by cultural norms and values in the culture of origin, which they have brought with them and pass to the next generation through social modelling. The most common example of this is the normalised use of (excessive) physical punishment. Ethnic minorities may hold onto these harmful behaviours for a range of reasons. For example, cultural norms are generally difficult to overturn anyway; cultural norms form the basis of cultural identity so changes to cultural norms are best to come from the inside (in line with the principle of 'self-determination') so as not to disrupt or displace sense of identity and belonging; cultural norms help new migrants have an 'anchor' or a reference point as they traverse the new culture, and cultural norms can become resistant to change when racism, discrimination and social exclusion are pronounced experiences for them: there is little motivation to integrate with a culture that makes them feel judged for who they are, and it interferes with the development of insight into their harmful parenting or a tendency to defend their harmful parenting.

Some harmful parenting by ethnic minorities is not determined by cultural norms, but instead by their need to adapt and settle into the new country. In this sense, harmful behaviours have arisen from 'acculturative' stress, related to factors like language barriers, social isolation, lack of extended family support and intergenerational conflict.

Some harmful behaviours by ethnic minority parents have nothing to do with culture or migration, and reflect 'generalist' issues that manifest among families of all groups regardless of their cultural background. These most often include domestic violence, alcohol or other drug issues and mental health issues in the carer.

Finally, some ethnic minority families enter the child protection system but have not necessarily behaved in a harmful way. The most common example of this is the tendency to label ethnic minorities as providing inadequate supervision to their children ('supervisory neglect'). This is an example of institutional racism.

If lack of awareness of this contextual story, and sensitivity and competency to address it in daily work practice, is sufficiently prevalent across caseworkers, management and systems, then this places ethnic minorities at risk of systematic disadvantage. At best, 'intervention within a family (should) not be inhibited or delayed by cultural considerations, (should) be moulded within a cultural framework in a way that makes the intervention meaningful and within the control of the family' (Giglio, 1997, p. 4), and should start where the client is (Zlotnik, 2007).

Knowledge of the story is best used to gain a contextualised understanding of a client family and where they may be coming from. Culture is but one part of the equation, and ethnic minorities do not want to be boxed, they just want to be understood. Overall, ethnic minorities have a continual pressure to both 'fit in' and 'be true to themselves' – this is their unique story. Failure to understand this compromises being able to provide a uniquely tailored service.

Equity: protecting cultural safety for all vulnerable groups to the same extent

Knowing when to celebrate cultural difference and at the same time acknowledge human sameness is a challenge in all multicultural, Western nations:

> *It's more important to look at the similarities between people rather than the differences. Diversity is important but people are more similar than they are different. [CW_ANON]*

While it is critical to appreciate what people across groups have in common, perhaps as a way of uniting them, there is a risk that structural disadvantages across groups are then minimised. For this reason, looking at differences between people and groups is also critical. When culture is not examined, it is at risk of being lost, and promoting and protecting the safety of cultures is essential to protecting children.

Cultural safety is equally at risk for all non-mainstream groups. However, this is not reflected in current institutional policies: mandatory consultation occurs for Indigenous families, but it does not occur for ethnic minorities. Thus, the need for cultural safety for ethnic minorities is less systemically acknowledged.

This may be reflective of broader politics regarding assimilation in Australia (and perhaps other Western countries). The severely costly lessons associated with attempts to overtly assimilate Indigenous Australians have been learned at the institutional level, leading to the practice of mandatory consultation. However, for ethnic minorities, political pressure in Australia still swings between 'multiculturalism' and 'assimilation', with Australian politicians undecided about what 'integration' looks like at the structural level.

For example, multiculturalism refers to (i) tolerance for, and/or acceptance of, people of different backgrounds or (ii) active government and institutional support for the recognition and acceptance of diverse ethnic identities and ancestries of the members of a society, also known as 'structural multiculturalism' (Koleth, 2010). The latter meaning is compromised by failing to make consultation with 'multicultural caseworkers' mandatory. Arguably, if Anglo Australians perceived themselves as migrants, they may be better able to acknowledge the importance of cultural preservation (instead of taking for granted their current ability to practise and preserve their culture), and which is not under threat of loss because of (hypothetical) pressure from original Indigenous landowners/custodians who expect them to assimilate to their way.

Thus, to promote equity, the ways in which the cultural needs of ethnic minorities are met need to be at least on par with ways made for Indigenous families. The most significant of these would be mandatory consultation.

In closing ...

There is a whole range of interactive and dynamic 'cultures' at play – the ethnic culture of the client family, the ethnic culture of the caseworker, 'Australian' culture, 'Western' culture and the organisational culture of child protection systems. Deep reflection on all of them, and the fact that the interaction between service users and service providers will always be racialised in the field, is required to best protect all children from harm equally.

Phillips (1995) notes that 'child abuse and protection are generally discussed from a framework of individual pathology rather than within the framework of inferiority-oppression and considering the politico-cultural and economic context of the group' (cited in Shalhoub-Kevorkian, 2005, p. 1266). 'The power of difference – particularly where one ethnic or racial group is considered inferior in customs, lifestyle, and beliefs – is a vital adjunct to the study of child protection' (Shalhoub-Kevorkian, 2005, p. 1266).

Similarly, Mason *et al.* (2002) say:

> Professionals who do not constructively engage with difference – and by this we mean from an assumption of equality and non-pathology – significantly lessen the chances of developing creative ways of working with people both within and across cultures. Engaging with difference enables us to explore the ties that bind and the ties that separate. Practitioners will then be enabled to develop cultural competency and thus play a positive role in eradicating racism and promoting and valuing diversity.
>
> (p. xxii)

With almost one-quarter of Australia's population born overseas and close to one-third from non-English speaking backgrounds (NESB), 'diversity is not a myth but a reality, and researchers, policy makers and service deliverers must strive to take it into account' (Weerasinghe and Williams, 2003, p. 8). In fact, Weerasinghe and Williams (2003) liken the need for ethnic diversity to be taken into account at the structural level, to that which preceded the feminist movement:

> It was not long ago that feminist scholars pushed to have gender recognised as an essential variable in all research, and today's efforts – encouraging a broad understanding of diversity – are somewhat analogous to those early days of the feminist movement ... 'diversity' cannot become marginalised as a subarea, but must become part of our perceived reality.
>
> (p. 8)

Although 'change is a slow process' (Chand, 2000, p. 76), it is a necessity. Indeed, the multicultural milieu of Australia and other Western countries will change in the future as different waves of migration occur, and as the number of children from mixed parentage increases (Katz, 1996; Barn, 1999). Above all, 'the opportunity of working in a multicultural society must be considered a privilege' (Koramoa *et al.*, 2002, p. 420), as it presents a unique opportunity for child protection agencies and practitioners to develop flexibly responsive policies and practices. And as awareness of cultural differences in parenting increases, child protection intervention will become more appropriate because the organisational and institutional knowledge and ability to respond to ethnic diversity will have improved; 'the novel will become normal'.

Future research

Westby (2007) notes that 'if intervention is to be appropriate and successful with immigrant children and families, professionals must be consistent in the messages they are giving' (p. 147). This book goes some way in meeting this need because it offers user-friendly models and resources that help promote consensus. Moreover, the practice and policy recommendations offered in this book are informed by the service users and service providers themselves. This is a demonstration of empowering the client group while developing an evidence-based framework of best practice for child protection work in a multicultural populace. Giving key stakeholders an inclusive and participatory voice improves the richness of the data: caseworkers and case managers are the frontline providers of child protection services and so are most aware of barriers to the effective implementation of culturally appropriate and sensitive service delivery, and ethnic minority families can identify the practices and policies they perceive or experience as in/effective in meeting their cultural needs. They also allow child protection staff to avoid 'repeating history's mistakes' and learn from the tried and tested local knowledge of other caseworkers:

> *It's just fantastic that you are doing this [research] because finally I get to say what I want done. [CW_NESB]*

Babacan (2006) notes that 'much of the literature is descriptive and there is very little work in terms of outcomes and what works at the intervention level' (p. 1). Again, this book goes some way in addressing the gap in knowledge by using robust and representative primary empirical data as the basis for evidence-based recommendations for good practice. Nevertheless, future research that empirically tests the rigour of these recommendations is still required to heed this call. Future research also helps expand the field and ensure that conversation about culture continues, and that complacency or tokenism does not threaten its importance:

> *I'm an oldie [in child protection] now, so we just remove, we don't have time to stop and think 'right, what do these kids need [culturally]'. [CW_NESB]*

Perhaps most importantly, however, future research needs to include and represent the voices of ethnic minority children themselves. While there are obvious limits to do with confidentiality and the need to adhere to child protection protocols (Williamson *et al.*, 2005), it is important their needs and experiences, and ideas for improving the cultural appropriateness of child protection service delivery, are captured and included when designing plans, policies and best practice models for this client group and their safety.

References

Ahmed, S. (2004). *Preventative services for Black and Minority Ethnic group children and families: A review of recent literature.* A paper for The National Evaluation of the Children's Fund, Birmingham.

Ali, S. (2006). Violence against the girl child in the Pacific Islands region. *UNICEF Innocenti Research Centre.* http://citeseerx.ist.psu.edu/viewdoc/download?doi=10.1.1.423.1594&rep=rep1&type=pdf

Al-Krenawi, A. and Graham, J. R. (2001). The cultural mediator: Bridging the gap between a non-Western community and professional social work practice. *British Journal of Social Work, 31,* 665–85.

Allport, G. (1979). *The nature of prejudice.* Reading, United Kingdom: Addison-Wesley.

Australian Bureau of Statistics (2007b). *Yearbook of Australia* (Cat. No. 1301.0). Canberra: Author.

Australian Bureau of Statistics (2007a). *Migration Australia* (Cat. No. 3412.0). Canberra: Author.

Australian Bureau of Statistics (2006b). *Population distribution, Aboriginal and Torres Strait Islander Australians* (Cat. No. 4705.0). Canberra: Author.

Australian Bureau of Statistics (2006a). *Experimental estimates and projections, Aboriginal and Torres Strait Islander Australians, 1991 to 2021* (Cat. No. 3238.0). Canberra: Author.

Australian Bureau of Statistics (2001). *The guide: Implementing the standards for statistics on cultural and language diversity.* Department of Immigration and Multicultural Affairs. Canberra: Author.

Babacan, H. (2006). *Literature review: Service/response models in child protection for culturally diverse communities.* Report prepared for the Department of Child Safety, Queensland.

Bagshaw, D. and Chung, D. (2001). The needs of children who witness domestic violence: A South Australian study. *Children Australia, 26(3),* 9–17.

Baker, P., Hussain, Z. and Saunders, J. (1991). *Interpreters in public services.* Birmingham: Venture Press.

Ban, P. and Swain, P. (1994). Family group conferences Part one: Australia's first project within child protection. *Children Australia, 19(3),* 19–21.

Barber, J. G., Delfabbro, P. H. and Cooper, L. (2000). Aboriginal and non-Aboriginal children in out of home care. *Children Australia, 25(3),* 5–10.

Barn, R. (2007). 'Race', ethnicity, and child welfare: A fine balancing act, Critical commentary. *British Journal of Social Work, 37(8),* 1–10.

Barn, R. (1999). White mothers, mixed-parentage children and child welfare. *British Journal of Social Work*, *29*, 269–84.

Barn, R., Sinclair, R. and Ferdinand, D. (1997). *Acting on principle: An examination of race and ethnicity in social services provision for children and families.* London: British Agencies for Adoption and Fostering.

Bartholet, E. (2009). Racial disproportionality movement in child welfare: False facts and dangerous directions, *Arizona Law Review*, *51*, 871–932.

Berry, J. W. (1980). Acculturation as varieties of adaptation. In A. M. Padilla (ed.), *Acculturation: Theory, models, and some new findings*. Boulder, CO: Westview.

Betts, K. (2002). Immigration and public opinion: Understanding this shift. *People & Place*, *10(4)*, 24–37.

Bond, M. H. (2002). Reclaiming the individual from Hofstede's ecological analysis: A 20 year odyssey. Comment on. *Psychological Bulletin, 128(1)*, 73–7.

Boushel, M. (2000). What kind of people are we? 'Race', anti-racism and social welfare research. *British Journal of Social Work*, *30(1)*, 71–89.

Brach, C. and Fraser, I. (2000). Can cultural competency reduce racial and ethnic health disparities? A review and conceptual model. *Medical Care Research & Review*, *57(Suppl. 1)*, 181–217.

Bromfield, L. and Arney, F. (2008). Developing a road map for research: Identifying priorities for a national child protection research agenda: Issues paper. *Australian Institute of Family Studies, No 28.*

Bromfield, L. and Holzer, P. (2008). Australian Institute of Family Studies Submission to the Special Commission of Inquiry into Child Protection Services in NSW. *Melbourne: Child Protection Clearinghouse, Australian Institute of Family Studies.*

Brophy, J., Jhutti-Johal, J. and McDonald, E. (2005). *Minority ethnic parents, their solicitors and child protection litigation.* Department for Constitutional Affairs.

Burke, S. and Paxman, M. (2008). *Children and young people from non-English speaking backgrounds in out of home care in NSW.* Sydney: NSW Department of Community Services.

Burton, L., Westen, D. and Kowalski, R. (2015). *Psychology: Australian and New Zealand edition* (4th edn). Milton, Australia: John Wiley and Sons.

Cahn, N. (2002). Race, poverty, history, adoption and child abuse: Connections. *Law & Society Review*, *36(2)*, 461–88.

Cashmore, J., Higgins, D. J., Bromfield, L. and Scott, D. A. (2006). Recent Australian child protection and out of home care research: What's been done and what needs to be done? *Children Australia, 31(2)*, 4–11.

Cazanave, N. A. and Maddern, D. A. (1999). Defending the white race: White male faculty opposition to a white racism course. *Race & Society*, *2*, 25–50.

Chan, J. S., Elliott, J. M., Chow, Y. and Thomas, J. I. (2002). Does professional and public opinion in child abuse differ? An issue of cross-cultural policy implementation. *Child Abuse Review*, *11*, 359–79.

Chand, A. (2005). Do you speak English? Language barriers in child protection social work with minority ethnic families. *British Journal of Social Work*, *35*, 807–21.

Chand, A. (2000). The over-representation of Black children in the child protection system: possible causes, consequences and solutions. *Child & Family Social Work, 5(1)*, 67–77.

Chand, A. and Thoburn, J. (2006). Research review: Child protection referrals and minority ethnic children and families. *Child & Family Social Work, 11*, 368–77.

Chand, A. and Thoburn, J. (2005). Research review: Child and family support services with minority ethnic families – what can we learn from research? *Child & Family Social Work, 10(2)*, 169–78.

Chang, J., Rhee, S. and Weaver, D. (2006). Characteristics of child abuse in immigrant Korean families and correlates of placement decisions. *Child Abuse & Neglect, 30*, 881–91.

Chin, W. Y. (2005). Blue spots, coining, and cupping: How ethnic minority parents can be misreported as child abusers. *Journal of Law in Society, 7(1)*, 88.

Choate, P. W. and Engstrom, S. (2014). The 'good enough' parent: Implications for child protection. *Child Care in Practice, 20(4)*, 368–82.

Chou, R. S. and Choi, S. (2013). And neither are we saved: Asian Americans' elusive quest for racial justice. *Sociology Compass, 7(10)*, 841–53.

Chuan, C. and Flynn, C. (2006). *Children and young people of culturally and linguistically diverse (CALD) backgrounds in out of home care in NSW: Support strategies, challenges, and issues: A qualitative research report*. Report prepared for Association of Children's Welfare Agencies (ACWA).

Clark, B. K. (1995). Acting in the best interest of the child: Essential components of a child custody evaluation. *Family Law Quarterly, 29(1)*, 19–38.

Cohan, J. A. (2010). *Apollonian and Dionysian cultures*. USA: Bentham E-books.

Connolly, M. (2007). Practice frameworks: Conceptual maps to guide interventions in child welfare. *British Journal of Social Work, 37(5)*, 825–37.

Connolly, M., Crichton-Hill, Y. and Ward, T. (2006). Culture and child protection: Reflexive responses. London, England: Jessica Kingsley Publishers.

Cousins, C. (2005). The 'rule of optimism': Dilemmas of embracing a strength-based approach in child protection work. *Children Australia, 30(2)*, 28–32.

Cowan, J. K., Dembour, M. and Wilson, R. A. (2001). *Culture and rights: Anthropological perspectives*. Cambridge: Cambridge University Press.

Crisante, L. (2005). Fiafia and ice-breaker morning tea: Parent education in Pacific Island communities. In Families Matter: 9th Australian Institute of Family Studies Conference, Melbourne Vic, February 2005 – proceedings.

Cross, T. L., Bazron, B. J., Dennis, K. W. and Isaacs, M. R. (1989). *Towards a culturally competent system of care: A monograph on effective services for minority children who are severely emotionally disturbed*. Washington, DC: CASSP Technical Assistance Center, Georgetown University Child Development Center.

Davidson, A. (1997). Multiculturalism and citizenship: Silencing the migrant voice. *Journal of Intercultural Studies, 18(2)*, 77–93.

Davidson, N., Skull, S., Burgner, D., Kelly, P., Raman, S., Silove, D., Steel, Z., Vora, R. and Smith, M. (2004). An issue of access: Delivering equitable health care for newly arrived refugee children in Australia. *Journal of Paediatric Child Health, 40(9–10)*, 569–75.

Dettlaff, A. J., Rivaux, S. L., Baumann, D. J., Fluke, J. D., Rycraft, J. R. and James, J. (2011). Disentangling substantiation: The influence of race, income, and risk on the substantiation decision in child welfare. *Children & Youth Services Review, 33(9)*, 1630–7.

Dewees, M. (2001). Building cultural competence for work with diverse families: Strategies from the privileged side. *Journal of Ethnic and Cultural Diversity in Social Work, 9(3/4)*, 33–51.

Dingwall, R., Eekelaar, J. and Murray, T. (2014). *The protection of children: State intervention and family life* (Vol. 16). Oxford: Quid Pro Books.

Dominelli, L. (1997). *Anti-racist social work* (2nd edn). Basingstoke: Macmillan Press.

Drake, B. and Jonson-Reid, M. (2011). NIS interpretations: Race and the national incidence studies of child abuse and neglect. *Children & Youth Services Review, 33(1)*, 16–20.

Dutt, R. and Phillips, M. (2000). Assessing black children in need and their families. In *Assessing children in need and their families: Practice guidance from the Department of Health*. London: The Stationery Office.

Elliott, A. and Sultman, C. (1998). Principles and processes for child protection decision-making: Queensland's case management framework. *Children Australia, 23(4)*, 9–14.

Elliott, B., Kiely, P. and Tolley, S. (2001). So much to gain: New approaches to child protection meetings. *Children Australia, 26(3)*, 23–6.

Elshaikh, Najet (1996). Working around the issue of access to NESB women, in *Many Voices, Different Stories*, Conference proceedings, Fairfield Multicultural Family Planning, Liverpool Printing Service, Sydney.

Ely, P. and Denney, D. (1987). *Social work in a multi-racial society*. Aldershot: Gower Publishing.

Evans, S., Huxley, P., Gately, C., Webber, M., Mears, A., Pajak, S., Medina, J., Kendall, T. and Katona, C. (2006). Mental health, burnout and job satisfaction among mental health social workers in England and Wales. *The British Journal of Psychiatry, 188(1)*, 75–80.

Feagin, J. R. and McKinney, K. D. (2003). *The many costs of racism*. Maryland: Rowman & Littlefield.

Featherstone, B., White, S. and Morris, K. (2014). *Re-imagining child protection: Towards humane social work with families*. Bristol: Policy Press.

Ferrari, A. M. (2002). The impact of culture upon child rearing practices and definitions of maltreatment. *Child Abuse & Neglect, 26(8)*, 793–813.

Fontes, L. A. (2005). *Child abuse and culture: Working with diverse families*. New York: Guilford Press.

Fontes, L. A. (2002). Child discipline and physical abuse in immigrant Latino families. *Journal of Counseling & Development, 80(1)*, 31–40.

Fontes, L. A. and Plummer, C. (2010). Cultural issues in disclosures of child sexual abuse. *Journal of Child Sexual Abuse, 19(5)*, 491–518.

Fontes, L., Cruz, M. and Tabachnick, J. (2001). Views of child sexual abuse in two cultural communities: An exploratory study among African Americans and Latinos. *Child Maltreatment, 6(2)*, 103–17.

Forehand, R. and Kotchick, B. A. (2002). Behavioural parent training: Current challenges and potential solutions. *Journal of Child & Family Studies, 11(4)*, 377–84.

Fraser, N. (2005). Reframing justice in a globalising world. *New Left Review, 36(Nov–Dec edn)*, 1–19.

Futa, K. T., Hsu, E. and Hansen, D. J. (2001). Child sexual abuse in Asian American families: An examination of cultural factors that influence prevalence, identification, and treatment. *Clinical Psychology: Science & Practice, 8(2)*, 189–209.

Gibbs, J. A. (2001). Maintaining front-line workers in child protection: A case for refocusing supervision. *Child Abuse Review, 10(5)*, 323–35.

Giglio, M. (1997). Child protection and cultural difference: Issues for NESB – non-English speaking background – communities. *Child Abuse Prevention, 5(2)*, 4–7.

Gilligan, P. and Akhtar, S. (2006). Cultural barriers to the disclosure of child sexual abuse in Asian communities: Listening to what women say. *British Journal of Social Work, 36(8)*, 1361–77.

Gillingham, P. (2006). Risk assessment in child protection: Problem rather than solution? *Australian Social Work, 59(1)*, 86–98.

Glaser, D. (2002). Emotional abuse and neglect (psychological maltreatment): A conceptual framework. *Child Abuse & Neglect, 26(6)*, 697–714.

Gleeson, J. P. (1995). Kinship care and public child welfare: Challenges and opportunities for social work education. *Journal of Social Work Education, 31*, 182–93.

Gonzalez, J. (2005). How to use an interpreter effectively. *Occupational Therapy Now, 7(2)*, 7–9.

Gordon, D. M., Oliveros, A., Hawes, S. W., Iwamoto, D. K. and Rayford, B. S. (2012). Engaging fathers in child protection services: A review of factors and strategies across ecological systems. *Children & Youth Services Review, 34(8)*, 1399–417.

Gough, D. and Lynch, M. A. (2002). Culture and child protection. *Child Abuse Review, 11*, 341–4.

Gray, B. (2003). Social exclusion, poverty, health and social care in Tower Hamlets: The perspectives of families on the impact of the family support service. *British Journal of Social Work, 33(3)*, 361–80.

Hackett, W. L. and Cahn, K. (2004). *Racial disproportionality in the child welfare system in King County, Washington*. Report prepared for King County Coalition on Racial Disproportionality.

Hage, G. (1998). Extract from 'White Nation: Fantasies of White supremacy in a multicultural society'. *People & Place, 7(1)*, 19–23.

Hahm, H. C. and Guterman, N. B. (2001). The emerging problem of physical child abuse in South Korea. *Child Maltreatment, 6*, 169–79.

Harran, E. (2002). Barriers to effective child protection in a multicultural society. *Child Abuse Review, 11(6)*, 411–14.

Harris, M. S. and Hackett, W. (2008). Decision points in child welfare: An action research model to address disproportionality. *Children & Youth Services Review, 30(2)*, 199–215.

Hawkins, M. F. and Briggs, F. (1999). Partnerships between parents and teachers in child protection. *Children Australia, 24(1)*, 8–13.

Healy, K., Meagher, G. and Cullin, J. (2009). Retaining novices to become expert child protection practitioners: Creating career pathways in direct practice. *British Journal of Social Work, 39(2)*, 299–317.

Hek, R. (2005). *The experiences and needs of refugee and asylum seeking children in the UK: A literature review*. A report for the National Evaluation of the Children's Fund. Research report RR 635.

Hesketh, T., Shu Hong, Z. and Lynch, M. A. (2000). Child abuse in China: The views and experiences of child health professionals. *Child Abuse & Neglect, 6(6)*, 867–72.

Hill, R. B. (2004). Institutional racism in child welfare. *Race & Society, 7(1)*, 17–33.

Hodgkin, S. (2002). Competing demands, competing solutions, differing constructions of the problem of recruitment and retention of frontline rural child protection staff. *Australian Social Work, 55(3)*, 193–203.

Hofstede, G. (2001). Culture's consequences: Comparing values, behaviors, institutions, and organizations across nations (2nd edn). Thousand Oaks, CA: Sage.

Hofstede, G. (1980). Culture's consequences: International differences in work-related values. Beverly Hills, CA: Sage.

Humphreys, C. (1999). Discrimination in child protection work: Recurring themes in work with Asian families. *Child and Family Social Work, 4*, 283–91.

Humphreys, C., Atkar, S. and Baldwin, N. (1999). Discrimination in child protection work: Recurring themes in work with Asian families. *Child and Family Social Work, 4*, 283–91.

Irfan, S. and Cowburn, M. (2004). Disciplining, chastisement, and physical child abuse: Perceptions and attitudes of the British Pakistani community. *Journal of Muslim Minority Affairs*, *24(1)*, 89–98.

Jackson, S. (1996). The kinship triad: A service delivery model. *Child Welfare*, *75*, 583–99.

Jackson, V. (2010). *Racism and child protection*. London: A&C Black.

Jent, J. F., Eaton, C. K., Knickerbocker, L., Lambert, W. F., Merrick, M. T. and Dandes, S. K. (2011). Multidisciplinary child protection decision making about physical abuse: Determining substantiation thresholds and biases. *Children & Youth Services Review*, *33(9)*, 1673–82.

Johnson, E. P., Clark, S., Donald, M., Pedersen, R. and Pichotta, C. (2007). Racial disparity in Minnesota's child protection system. *Child Welfare*, *86(4)*, 5–20.

Kanuha, V. (1994). Women of color in battering relationships. In Comas-Diaz, L. and Greene, B. (eds), *Women of color: Integrating ethnic and gender identities in psychotherapy*. New York: Guilford, pp. 428–54.

Katerndahl, D., Burge, S., Kellogg, N. and Parra, J. (2005). Differences in childhood sexual abuse experience between adult Hispanic and Anglo women in a primary care setting. *Journal of Child Sexual Abuse*, *14(2)*, 85–95.

Katz, I. (1996). *The construction of racial identity in children of mixed parentage – mixed metaphors*. London: Jessica Kingsley Publishers.

Kaur, J. (2007). Working with families from culturally and linguistically diverse communities in Queensland: An Australian exploratory study. *Children Australia*, *32(4)*, 17–24.

Kim, H., Chenot, D. and Ji, J. (2011). Racial/ethnic disparity in child welfare systems: A longitudinal study utilizing the Disparity Index (DI). *Children & Youth Services Review*, *33(7)*, 1234–44.

Kim, I. J., Lau, A. S. and Chang, D. F. (2006). Family violence among Asian Americans. In *Social and Personal Adjustment*, pp. 364–78. www.aasc.ucla.edu/policy/kim_lau_chang.pdf

Koleth, E. (2010). *Multiculturalism: A review of Australian policy statements and recent debates in Australia and overseas*. Research Paper No. 6, Parliament of Australia.

Koramoa, J., Lynch, M. A. and Kinnair, D. (2002). A continuum of child-rearing: Responding to traditional practices. *Child Abuse Review*, *11(6)*, 415–21.

Korbin, J. (2008). Child neglect and abuse across cultures. In Robinson, G., Eickelkamp, U., Goodnow, J. and Katz, I. (eds), *Contexts of child development culture, policy and intervention*. Darwin: Charles Darwin University Press, pp. 122–30.

Korbin, J. E. (2002). Culture and child maltreatment: Cultural competence and beyond. *Child Abuse & Neglect*, *26(6)*, 637–44.

Krane, J., Davies, L., Carlton, R. and Mulcahy, M. (2010). The clock starts now: Feminism, mothering and attachment theory in child protection practice. In Featherstone, B., Hooper, C., Scourfield, J. and Taylor, J. (eds), *Gender & child welfare in society*. Wiley-Blackwell: West Sussex, UK, pp. 149–72.

Križ, K. and Skivenes, M. (2012). Child-centric or family focused? A study of child welfare workers' perceptions of ethnic minority children in England and Norway. *Child & Family Social Work*, *17(4)*, 448–57.

Križ, K. and Skivenes, M. (2011). How child welfare workers view their work with racial and ethnic minority families: The United States in contrast to England and Norway. *Children & Youth Services Review*, *33(10)*, 1866–74.

Križ, K. and Skivenes, M. (2010). Lost in translation: How child welfare workers in Norway and England experience language difficulties when working with minority ethnic families. *British Journal of Social Work, 40(5)*, 1353–67.

Križ, K., Slayter, E., Iannicelli, A. and Lourie, J. (2012). Fear management: How child protection workers engage with non-citizen immigrant families. *Children & Youth Services Review, 34(1)*, 316–23.

Krizsán, A. (2001). *Ethnic monitoring and data protection: The European context.* Budapest, Hungary: Central European University Press.

Lau, J. T. F., Liu, J. L. Y., Yu, A. and Wong, C. K. (1999). Conceptualisation, reporting and underreporting of child abuse in Hong Kong. *Child Abuse & Neglect, 23(11)*, 1159–74.

Lee, M. Y. and Greene, G. J. (2003). A teaching framework for transformative multicultural social work education. *Journal of Ethnic and Cultural Diversity in Social Work, 12(3)*, 1–28.

Lemon, K., D'Andrade, A. and Austin, M. J. (2005). *Understanding and addressing disproportionality in the front end of the child welfare system.* California: Centre of Social Services Research.

Lenette, C., Brough, M. and Cox, L. (2013). Everyday resilience: Narratives of single refugee women with children. *Qualitative Social Work, 12(5)*, 637–53.

Lu, Y. E., Landsverk, J., Ellis-Macleod, E., Newton, R., Ganger, W. and Johnson, I. (2004). Race, ethnicity, and case outcomes in child protective services. *Children & Youth Services Review, 26(5)*, 447–61.

McConnell, D. and Llewellyn, G. (2005). Social inequality, 'the deviant parent' and child protection practice. *Australian Journal of Social Issues, 40(4)*, 553–66.

McPhatter, A. R. (1997). Cultural competence in child welfare: What is it? How do we achieve it? What happens without it? *Child Welfare, 76(1)*, 225–78.

Maiter, S. and Stalker, C. (2011). South Asian immigrants' experience of child protection services: Are we recognizing strengths and resilience? *Child & Family Social Work, 16(2)*, 138–48.

Maiter, S., Alaggia, R. and Trocmé, N. (2004). Perceptions of child maltreatment by parents from the Indian subcontinent: Challenging myths about culturally based abusive parenting practices. *Child Maltreatment, 9(3)*, 309–24.

Maitra, B. (2005). Culture and child protection. *Current Paediatrics, 15(3)*, 253–9.

Makhoul, J., Ghanem, D. S. and Ghanem, M. (2003). An ethnographic study of the consequences of social and structural forces on children: The cause of two low-income Beirut suburbs. *Environment & Urbanisation, 15(2)*, 249–59.

Mansell, J., Ota, R., Erasmus, R. and Marks, K. (2011). Reframing child protection: A response to a constant crisis of confidence in child protection. *Children & Youth Services Review, 33(11)*, 2076–86.

Marie, D., Fergusson, D. M. and Boden, J. M. (2009). Ethnic identity and exposure to maltreatment in childhood: Evidence from a New Zealand Birth Cohort. *Social Policy Journal of New Zealand, 36(36)*, 154–71.

Markward, M., Dozier, C., Hooks, K. and Markward, N. (2000). Culture and the intergenerational transmission of substance abuse, woman abuse, and child abuse: A diathesis–stress perspective. *Children & Youth Services Review, 22(3)*, 237–50.

Mason, B., Sawyer, A. and Boyd-Franklin, N. (2002). *Exploring the unsaid: Creativity, risks, and dilemmas in working cross-culturally.* London: Karnac Books.

Mendes, P. (1999). Marxist and feminist critiques of child protection: To protect children or to change society? *Children Australia, 24(2)*, 27–31.

Mildred, J. and Plummer, C. A. (2009). Responding to child sexual abuse in the United States and Kenya: Child protection and children's rights. *Children & Youth Services Review, 31(6)*, 601–8.

Miller, A. B. and Cross, T. (2006). Ethnicity in child maltreatment research: A replication of Behl *et al.*'s content analysis. *Child Maltreatment, 11(1)*, 16–26.

Missingham, B., Dibden, J. and Cocklin, C. (2006). A multicultural countryside? Ethnic minorities in rural Australia. *Rural Society, 16(2)*, 131–50.

Munro, E. (2010). Learning to reduce risk in child protection. *British Journal of Social Work, 40(4)*, 1135–51.

Munro, E. (2005). Improving practice: Child protection as a systems problem. *Children & Youth Services Review, 27(4)*, 375–91.

Munro, E. (2004). A simpler way to understand the results of risk assessment instruments. *Children & Youth Services Review, 26(9)*, 873–83.

Munro E. (1996). Avoidable and unavoidable mistakes in child protection work. *British Journal of Social Work, 26*, 795–810.

Nybell, L. M. and Gray, S. S. (2004). Race, place and space: Meanings of cultural competence in three child welfare agencies. *Social Work, 49(1)*, 17–26.

O'Hagan, K. (1999). Culture, cultural identity, and cultural sensitivity in child and family social work. *Child & Family Social Work, 4(4)*, 269–81.

O'Leary, P., Coohey, C. and Easton, S. D. (2010). The effect of severe child sexual abuse and disclosure on mental health during adulthood. *Journal of Child Sexual Abuse, 19(3)*, 275–89.

Omar, Y. (2005). Young Somalis in Australia: An educational approach to challenges and recommended solutions. *Migration Action, 27(1)*, 6–18.

O'Neale, V. (2000). *Excellence not excuses: Inspection of services for ethnic minority children and families*. London: Social Services Inspectorate.

O'Neil, D. (2005). How can a strengths approach increase safety in a child protection context? *Children Australia, 30(4)*, 28–32.

O'Shaughnessy, R., Collins, C. and Fatimilehin, I. (2010). Building bridges in Liverpool: Exploring the use of Family Group Conferences for black and minority ethnic children and their families. *British Journal of Social Work, 40(7)*, 2034–49.

Osofsky, J. D. (2003). Prevalence of children's exposure to domestic violence and child maltreatment: Implications for prevention and intervention. *Clinical Child & Family Psychology Review, 6(3)*, 161–70.

Owen, M. and Farmer, E. (1996). Child protection in a multi-racial context. *Policy and Politics, 24*, 299–313.

Owusu-Bempah, K. (1999). Race, culture and the child. In J. Tunstill (ed.), *Children and the state: Whose problem?* London: Cassell.

Papps, E. and Ramsden, I. (1996). Cultural safety in nursing: The New Zealand experience. *International Journal for Quality in Health Care, 8(5)*, 491–7.

Parkinson, P. (2003). Child protection, permanency planning and children's right to family life. *International Journal of Law, Policy and the Family, 17(2)*, 147–72.

Parton, N. (2009). How child centred are our child protection systems and how child centred do we want our child protection regulatory principles to be? *Communities, Children & Families Australia, 4(1)*, 59–64.

Pedersen, P. (1989). Developing multicultural ethics guidelines for psychology. *International Journal of Psychology, 24(5)*, 643–52.

Pelczarski, Y. and Kemp, S. P. (2006). Patterns of child maltreatment referrals among Asian and Pacific Islander families. *Child Welfare, 85(1)*, 5–31.

Perry, R. and Limb, G. E. (2004). Ethnic/racial matching of clients and social workers in public child welfare. *Children & Youth Services Review, 26(10)*, 965–79.

Phillips, M. (1995). Issues of ethnicity and culture. In K. Wilson and A. L. James (eds), *The child protection handbook*. London: Balliare Tindall, pp. 108–25.

Pinderhughes, E. E. (1991). The delivery of child welfare services to African American clients. *American Journal of Orthopsychiatry, 61(4)*, 599–605.

Qiao, D. P. and Chan, Y. C. (2005). Child abuse in China: A yet-to-be-acknowledged 'social problem' in the Chinese Mainland. *Child & Family Social Work, 10(1)*, 21–7.

Radford, L., Corral, S., Bradley, C., Fisher, H., Bassett, C., Howat, N. and Collishaw, S. (2011). *Child abuse and neglect in the UK today.* London: NSPCC. www.nspcc.org.uk/childstudy

Raman, S. and Hodes, D. (2012). Cultural issues in child maltreatment. *Journal of Paediatrics & Child Health, 48(1)*, 30–7.

Rapoza, K. A., Cook, K., Zaveri, T. and Malley-Morrison, K. (2010). Ethnic perspectives on sibling abuse in the United States. *Journal of Family Issues, 31(6)*, 808–29.

Reisig, J. A. and Miller, M. K. (2009). How the social construction of 'child abuse' affects immigrant parents: Policy changes that protect children and families. *International Journal of Social Inquiry, 2(1)*, 17–37.

Roberts, D. E. (2008). The racial geography of child welfare: Toward a new research paradigm. *Child Welfare, 87(2)*, 125–50.

Roberts, D. E. (2003). Child welfare and civil rights. *University of Illinois Review, 1*, 171–82.

Roberts, D. E. (1997). *Killing the black body: Race, reproduction, and the meaning of liberty.* New York: Pantheon Books.

Russell, M. N. and White, B. (2001). Practice with immigrant and refugees: Social worker and client perspectives. *Journal of Ethnic and Cultural Diversity in Social Work, 9(3/4)*, 73–92.

Sale, A. U. (2006). Paralysed around culture. *Community Care, 1614*, 28–9.

Sandau-Beckler, P., Salcido, R., Beckler, M. J., Mannes, M. and Beck, M. (2002). Infusing family-centered values into child protection practice. *Children & Youth Services Review, 24(9–10)*, 719–41.

Satzewich, V. (1998). *Racism and social inequality in Canada: Concepts, controversies and strategies of resistance.* Toronto: Thompson Educational Publishing.

Sawrikar, P. (2010c). *Final Report – Culturally appropriate service provision for culturally and linguistically diverse (CALD) children and families in the New South Wales (NSW) child protection system.* Sydney: NSW Department of Community Services. www.sprc.unsw.edu.au/media/SPRCFile/17_CALD_families_in_CPS_Final_Report.pdf

Sawrikar, P. (2010b). *Interim Report 3 – Culturally appropriate service provision for culturally and linguistically diverse (CALD) children and families in the New South Wales (NSW) child protection system: qualitative interviews with CALD families and caseworkers.* Sydney: NSW Department of Community Services. www.sprc.unsw.edu.au/media/SPRCFile/18_CALD_families_in_CPS_Interim_Report_3.pdf

Sawrikar, P. (2010a). *Interim Report 2 – Culturally appropriate service provision for culturally and linguistically diverse (CALD) children and families in the New South Wales (NSW) child protection system: Case file review.* Sydney: NSW Department of Community Services. www.sprc.unsw.edu.au/media/SPRCFile/19_CALD_families_in_CPS_Interim_Report_2.pdf

Sawrikar, P. (2009). *Interim Report 1 – Culturally appropriate service provision for culturally and linguistically diverse (CALD) children and families in the New South*

Wales (NSW) child protection system: Literature review. Sydney: NSW Department of Community Services. www.sprc.unsw.edu.au/media/SPRCFile/20_Report_Cald_Families _LitRvw.pdf

Sawrikar, P. and Hunt, C. (2005). The relationship between mental health, cultural identity, and cultural values, in non-English speaking background (NESB) Australian adolescents, *Behaviour Change, 22(2)*, 97–113.

Sawrikar, P. and Katz, I. (2010). "Only White people can be racist": What does power have to do with prejudice? *Cosmopolitan Civil Societies, 2(1)*, 80–99.

Sawrikar, P. and Katz, I. (2009). *How useful is the term Culturally and Linguistically Diverse (CALD) in the Australian social policy discourse?* Refereed Conference Paper, Australian Social Policy Conference, July 2009, Sydney. www.aspc.unsw.edu.au/sites/ www.aspc.unsw.edu.au/files/uploads/aspc_historical_conferences/2009/paper276.pdf

Sawrikar, P. and Katz, I. (2008). *Enhancing family and relationship service accessibility and delivery to culturally and linguistically diverse families in Australia*. Australia Family Relationships Clearinghouse, *Issue No. 3*. www.sprc.unsw.edu.au/media/SPRC File/3_Report_AFRC_Issues3.pdf

Sawrikar, P., Griffiths, M. and Muir, K. (2008). *Culturally and Linguistically Diverse (CALD) young people and mentoring: The case of Horn of African young people in Australia*. Report to the National Youth Affairs Research Scheme (NYARS). www. sprc.unsw.edu.au/media/SPRCFile/40_Report_NYARS_CALD_Nov08.pdf

Selwyn, J. and Wijedesa, D. (2011). Pathways to adoption for minority ethnic children in England – reasons for entry to care. *Child & Family Social Work, 16(3)*, 276–86.

Seth, R. and Raman, S. (2014). What do we know about child neglect? A global perspective. In Conte, J. (ed.), *Child abuse and neglect worldwide*. California: Praeger, pp. 123–53.

Shalhoub-Kevorkian, N. (2005). Disclosure of child abuse in conflict areas. *Violence Against Women, 11(10)*, 1263–91.

Sidebotham, P. (2013). Authoritative child protection. *Child Abuse Review, 22(1)*, 1–4.

Sidebotham, P. and Heron, J. (2006). Child maltreatment in the 'children of the nineties': A cohort study of risk factors. *Child Abuse & Neglect, 30(5)*, 497–522.

Sinclair, K. (1995). Responding to abuse: A matter of perspective. *Current Issues in Criminal Justice, 7(2)*, 153–75.

Singh, G. (1992). *Race and social work: From 'black pathology' to 'black perspectives'*. Race Relations Research Unit, Bradford.

Slack, K. S., Holl, J. L., McDaniel, M., Yoo, J. and Bolger, K. (2004). Understanding the risks of child neglect: An exploration of poverty and parenting characteristics. *Child Maltreatment, 9(4)*, 395–408.

So-Kum Tang, C. (1998). The rate of physical child abuse in Chinese families: A community survey in Hong Kong. *Child Abuse & Neglect, 22(5)*, 381–91.

Starbuck, E. (1994). Competency – views from one child protection front. *Children Australia, 19(2)*, 27–30.

Stokes, J. and Schmidt, G. (2011). Race, poverty and child protection decision making. *British Journal of Social Work, 41(6)*, 1105–21.

Suaalii, T. M. and Mavoa, H. (2001). Who says yes? Collective and individual framing of Pacific children's consent to, and participation in, research in New Zealand. *Childrenz Issues, 5(1)*, 39–42.

Taylor, J. (2004). Refugees and social exclusion: What the literature says. *Migration Action, 26(2)*, 16–31.

Thanki, V. (2007). Ethnic diversity and child protection. *Children & Society, 8(3)*, 232–44.

Thoburn, J., Chand, A. and Procter, J. (2005). *Child welfare services for minority ethnic families: The research reviewed.* London: Jessica Kingsley Publishers.

Thom, N. (2008). Using telephone interpreters to communicate with patients. *Nursing Times, 104(46),* 28–9.

Thomson, D. M. and Molloy, S. E. (2001). Assessing the best interests of the child. *The Australian Educational & Developmental Psychologist, 18(2),* 5–14.

Thorpe, R. (2007). Family inclusion in child protection practice: Building bridges in working with (not against) families. *Communities, Children & Families Australia, 3(1),* 4.

Tilbury, C. (2006). Accountability via performance measurement: The case of Child Protection Services. *Australian Journal of Public Administration, 65(3),* 48–61.

Tomison, A. M. (2001). A history of child protection: Back to the future? *Family Matters, 60(60),* 46–57.

Triandis, H. C. (1990). Theoretical concepts that are applicable to the analysis of ethnocentricism. In Brislin, R. W. (ed.), *Applied cross-cultural psychology.* New York: Sage, pp. 34–55.

Trocmé, N., Knoke, D. and Blackstock, C. (2004). Pathways to the overrepresentation of Aboriginal children in Canada's child welfare system. *Social Service Review, 78(4),* 577–600.

Trogan, I., Dessypris, N., Moustaki, M. and Petridou, E. (2001). How common is abuse in Greece? Studying cases with femoral fractures. *Archives of Disease in Childhood, 85(4),* 289–92.

Trotter, C. and Sheehan, R. (2000). Family group conferencing: An evaluation. *Children Australia, 25(4),* 37–41.

Tufford, L., Bogo, M. and Asakura, K. (2015). How do social workers respond to potential child neglect? *Social Work Education, 34(2),* 229–43.

Vaughan, G. M. and Hogg, M. A. (2002). *Introduction to social psychology* (3rd edn). London: Prentice Hall.

Walker, S. (2002). Culturally competent protection of children's mental health. *Child Abuse Review, 11(6),* 380–93.

Ward, B. M., Anderson, K. S. and Sheldon, M. S. (2005). Patterns of home and community care service delivery to culturally and linguistically diverse residents of rural Victoria. *Australian Journal of Rural Health, 13(6),* 348–52.

Webb, E., Maddocks, A. and Bongilli, J. (2002). Effectively protecting Black and Minority ethnic children from harm: Overcoming barriers to the child protection process. *Child Abuse Review, 11(6),* 394–410.

Weerasinghe, S. and Williams, L. S. (2003). Health and the intersections of diversity: A challenge paper on selected program, policy and research issues. In *Intersections of Diversity Seminar,* Niagara Falls, Canada.

Welbourne, P. (2002). Culture, children's rights and child protection. *Child Abuse Review, 11(6),* 345–58.

Westby, C. E. (2007). Child maltreatment: A global issue. *Language, Speech & Hearing Services in Schools, 38(2),* 140–8.

Whittaker, A. (2011). Social defences and organisational culture in a local authority child protection setting: Challenges for the Munro Review? *Journal of Social Work Practice, 25(4),* 481–95.

Wilhelmus, M. (1998). Mediation in kinship care: Another step in the provision of culturally relevant child welfare services. *Social Work, 43(2),* 117–26.

Wilkins, D. (2012). Disorganised attachment indicates child maltreatment: How is this link useful for child protection social workers? *Journal of Social Work Practice, 26(1),* 15–30.

Williams, C. and Soydan, H. (2005). When and how does ethnicity matter? A cross-national study of social work responses to ethnicity in child protection cases. *British Journal of Social Work, 35(6),* 901–20.

Williams, N. (2008). Refugee participation in South Australian child protection research: Power, voice, and representation. *Family & Consumer Sciences Research Journal, 37(2),* 191–209.

Williamson, E., Goodenough, T., Kent, J. and Ashcroft, R. (2005). Conducting research with children: The limits of confidentiality and child protection protocols. *Children & Society, 19(5),* 397–409.

Winkworth, G. and McArthur, M. (2006). Being 'child-centred' in child protection: What does it mean? *Children Australia, 31(4),* 13–21.

Wilson, M. (1993). *Crossing the boundary.* London: Virago.

Wurtzburg, S. J. (2000). The Domestic Violence Act, gender, and ethnicity: Pacific Island people in Christchurch, New Zealand. *Development Bulletin, 51,* 26–9.

Yick, A. G. (2007). Role of culture and context: Ethical issues in research with Asian Americans and immigrants in intimate violence. *Journal of Family Violence, 22(5),* 277–85.

Zanoni, L., Warburton, W., Bussey, K. and McMaugh, A. (2014). Are all fathers in child protection families uncommitted, uninvolved and unable to change? *Children & Youth Services Review, 41,* 83–94.

Zlotnik, J. L. (2007). Evidence-based practice and social work education: A view from Washington. *Research on Social Work Practice, 17(5),* 625–9.

Index